"Most journalists are intimidated by science. . . . The consequences for a journalist in getting it wrong in covering a political issue, or a sporting event, or a business development amount to embarrassment. Getting it wrong in vaccines, and possibly being responsible for the death or disability of innocents, involves taking on more responsibility than many journalists can countenance. Even if the journalist doesn't get it wrong, in the absence of proof, he will be blamed as if he did, making him a pariah. Again, this isn't the role that journalists want for themselves."—Lawrence Solomon, columnist for the National Post, former a columnist for the *Globe and Mail*, contributor to the *Wall Street Journal* and publisher of the award-winning *The Next City* magazine.

"The mainstream media treats the peer-reviewed scientific literature as if it's uncorrupted by special interests. Nothing could be further from the truth. Scientists and the institutions where they work are just as subject to corruption as Congress, the Catholic Church, and any other institution run by human beings, including the mainstream media itself."—David Lewis, PhD, former senior-level research microbiologist at the US EPA Office of Research & Development

"In the 1980s and 90s, US journalists examined and reported on legitimate questions about gaps in vaccine safety science, one-size-fits all vaccine policies, and conflicts of interest between Big Pharma, medical trade, and public health agencies. Although in the twenty-first century too many old guard media outlets simply reprint government and industry press releases, there is a robust public conversation about vaccination and health taking place on the Internet and parents of vaccine injured children are at the forefront of that important conversation."—Barbara Loe Fisher, vaccine safety advocate

"The media has been used to influence opinion at all levels—from the judiciary and political leaders, to the man and woman on the street. And turned on in critical moments, for example, displacing blame for vaccine failures during disease outbreaks. For those at street level in particular, its false message has failed miserably. Why? Because 33 percent of US parents with children under 18 believe vaccines cause autism. Why? Because the truth is in plain sight every day, on every street, in every school. Not because of one man or one celebrity. A measure of the integrity of the media—what is left of it—will be its reaction when forced to face the fact that it is a whore."—Andrew Wakefield, MD

"As citizens of this capitalist nation, we cannot rely on corporate-sponsored news media for the truth."—Kelly Brogan, MD, Holistic Women's Health Psychiatry, New York, NY

# THE BIG AUTISM COVER-UP

# THE BIG AUTISM COVER-UP

## HOW AND WHY THE MEDIA IS LYING TO THE AMERICAN PUBLIC

ANNE DACHEL

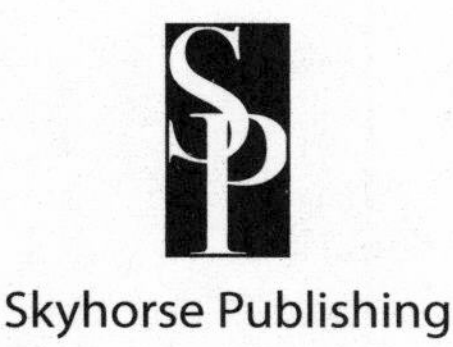


Skyhorse Publishing

Skyhorse Publishing books may be purchased in bulk at special discounts for sales promotion, corporate gifts, fund-raising, or educational purposes. Special editions can also be created to specifications. For details, contact the Special Sales Department, Skyhorse Publishing, 307 West 36th Street, 11th Floor, New York, NY 10018 or info@skyhorsepublishing.com.



Visit our website at www.skyhorsepublishing.com.

10 9 8 7 6 5 4 3 2 1

Library of Congress Cataloging-in-Publication Data is available on file.

Cover design by Danielle Ceccolini

Print ISBN: 978-1-62914-446-7
Ebook ISBN: 978-1-62914-870-0

Printed in the United States of America

To my beloved husband, Richard, for his constant support.

To my children, John, Catherine, Laura and Daniel, for putting up with my hours on the computer.

To my wonderful aunt, Dolores Logan, for all the encouraging conversations.

Special recognition to the four outstanding journalists who have dared to honestly and thoroughly cover this controversy: David Kirby, Dan Olmsted, Sharyl Attkisson, and Alisyn Camerota.

# Contents

*"If you want to sell a lie, get the press to sell it for you."*

—*Argo*, 2012

*"The two most misguided notions held in America: Our government wouldn't really do that to us; if they did, they would tell us about it on TV."*

—Anonymous

*"Oh my God, I cannot believe we did what we did, but we did. It's the lowest point in my career, that I went along with that paper. I went along with this, we didn't report significant findings. . . . I have great shame now when I meet families with kids with autism because I have been part of the problem. . . . I was complicit and I went along with this. . . . We didn't report significant findings. . . . The higher-ups wanted to do certain things, and I went along with it."*

—Dr. William Thompson, August, 2014
Senior CDC scientist breaking thirteen years of silence on the CDC study that found an increased risk of autism in African American boys receiving the MMR vaccine on time compared with those receiving it later.

# Foreword

## Autism as a Symptom of Our Dystopia

I wanted to write this for Anne's book because it has been and continues to be such an honor to know her and work with her. We have coauthored several articles, such as our first, "Throwing Children into Oncoming Traffic." (2007)

Anne has been an unsung truth-teller, unrelenting in her Internet commentaries about what the media is prevaricating about from one day to the next as it relates to what autism is doing to our children. A daunting task for one human, but she has been at it now for years and has never missed a beat.

You will discern this for yourself as you read the pages of this revealing book about a seriously troubling subject that makes me often ashamed to be a physician. In our "modern times," we have almost no concept of our true present, let alone our true past. Neither do we grasp our vulnerability as humans on this planet.

Let me take you back to the year 1989, when the first child with "autism" that I had ever laid eyes on was brought into my office by his mother. I did not know it was autism at first as I had not been taught anything about autism in medical school and had never encountered a child with autism through my residency at UCLA. I studied this four-year-old boy carefully. I could see intelligence behind his eyes but an increasingly high level of frustration was building as it was clear he was trying to communicate verbally and nothing intelligent would come from his lips, just like an old-time phone switchboard where all the wrong wires were plugged into all the wrong connections. The frustration overwhelmed him, and he lost his composure.

I remember going through textbooks later that day thinking I had just seen 1 in 10,000. I had been a board-certified pediatrician for more than two decades, and I can tell you these kids were not there at the beginning of the last quarter of the twentieth century. I saw a lot of rare and unusual disorders, but I had never seen a case of autism before that day.

Yet, HHS, the CDC, and NIMH would have us all believe that pediatricians who practiced in the seventies and eighties were not astute enough to diagnose autism, that these children and adults were among us all the time, and that we just "missed" all these little people who would suddenly stop talking, become incontinent, scream all day, walk on their toes, and throw themselves on the floor in supermarkets and parking lots when they weren't just trying to run off without direction or purpose.

Any illness that goes from 1 in 10,000 to 1 in 50 in the course of a couple of decades should be of interest to members of the media but, sadly, they're content to merely repeat the tired claims of health officials and leave every aspect of autism as one big mystery.

Why aren't members of the media looking for all those autistic adults that we called something else before we became so enlightened?

Instead, why are we told over and over that all the autism is nothing new and that it isn't really a problem society needs to concern itself with? Is autism called a genetic disorder because then no one need be concerned about the cause because it's something kids are born with?

If we want the situation to change, we have to stop lying to ourselves about it first and foremost. We may not be able to control who lies to us, but the media shouldn't be repeating the lies, unquestioned. That is the first step, so let's start there.

When I talk to the parents of affected children, a very large percentage of them are not mystified by what happened to their children. They know what caused them to develop autism. It was the vaccinations their child received.

In the last decade, I have lost count of how many hundreds of affected children I have treated. It is often a multisystem disorder, with several comorbid infections, allergies, gut issues, endocrine abnormalities, and toxic burdens. Not everyone recovers, nor is everyone recoverable, but much can be done for many if we can stop all the prevarication about what is causing the chronic disease around us.

It has been ten years since I was invited to give testimony in front of the House Committee on Government Reform and Oversight (Health Subcommittee) by US Congressman Dan Burton of Indiana. At that time, a few members of Congress were truly interested in what could be done for all the Autism Spectrum Disorder children. I naively thought something would come from this, but two years later, a congressional staffer who had been at that hearing told me there would never be a bill passed in Congress that had the words "autism" and "treatment" in it.

Congress wasn't interested in really helping children disabled with autism.

At that time, I was about to propose a constructive plan to have affected children treated, but "treatment" means there is something to treat, which also means there is a reason there is something to be treated. So nothing has happened to help affected children, and nothing has been done to understand the cause. Instead, it is politically correct to say autism is a genetic disorder kids are born with. Analysis of the funding shows it is all directed at trying to find that elusive genetic cause. Never mind there has never been a genetic epidemic. We have wasted millions of dollars on gene research while doing nothing to stop an epidemic.

News reports flood the public with confusing and contradictory stories about autism and its possible cause. What the media doesn't cover is the fact that today more and more scientists are recognizing that environmental toxins are strongly implicated in the autism epidemic. Sadly, even many of the people who recognize that toxic chemicals cause autism are unwilling to link autism to the toxins we regularly inject into children in their vaccines.

Incredibly, courses in environmental and nutritional medicine are not taught in medical schools, despite the fact that the greatest strides in human health have taken place because of improvements in sanitation and proper nutrition. These subjects are not taught because they have nothing to do with promoting and selling patented medicines.

And a child who develops autism has that genetic disposition to be severely affected by the onslaught of toxic exposures in the environment.

Autism is an environmentally triggered immunoencephalopathy (a disease of the brain caused by something in the environment and which engages the immune system) that is often mediated by mitochondrial dysfunction. And because there are triggers, it can potentially be treated by removing the toxins and repairing the damage.

It is past the time to recognize what is happening to our children.

—Kenneth Stoller, MD

# Introduction

On September 19, 2012, Kim Stagliano, author of *All I Can Handle: I'm No Mother Teresa: A Life Raising Three Daughters with Autism*, was on *Good Morning Texas* at WFAA in Dallas. As she talked, family photos appeared showing her three daughters, all of whom have autism. The conversation focused on the problems parents face and the need for services for what Stagliano called "an epidemic." The reporter interviewing Kim at WFAA said that she herself had a child on the autism spectrum. She asked Kim why news outlets weren't talking about autism as a crisis. Kim answered, "I don't know, but there has been a concerted effort across the media to play down the tragedy of the epidemic. These are children who may never live up to their full potential. Part of my work is to raise that alarm bell that we need to do more."

During the course of the interview, Stagliano mentioned that she was in Dallas to attend a luncheon for workers "who service over 60,000 children in Dallas County who have developmental disabilities." She said that she hoped research would tell us how to prevent autism, something rarely ever mentioned in autism stories in the news.

This interview on WFAA asked the really important question about why members of the media cover autism like they do. Why doesn't the press report on autism as a serious health care issue? Why don't we see words like "crisis" and "epidemic" in stories about autism?

Members of the media have consistently backed the people who are out to convince us that autism is a normal and acceptable part of childhood. Every stunning increase in the autism rate is presented as merely "better diagnosing" and no real increase. On a regular basis, studies are publicized linking autism to genetics or the actions of parents. We don't see the severe side of autism in the two-minute news coverage of walks for awareness or autism fundraisers. Despite all the evidence to the contrary, news stories universally reassure us that there is no link between autism and the ever-expanding vaccine schedule and pit misguided parents and debunked research up against the medical community and health officials. No one in the mainstream media is ever worried about the fact that when we talk about autism, we're almost always talking about children with autism. No one wonders why we have to train teachers, firefighters, EMTs, and police to deal with individuals with autism. No one asks why we have to have "sensory friendly" movie showings and "sensitive Santas" and "autism friendly" story times at the library. No one looks for the misdiagnosed or undiagnosed adults in group homes and institutions in order to give us the proof that autism has always been around at the rate we see in our children. No one questions the motives of the agency that runs the vaccine program when they produce yet another study showing their vaccines don't harm children.

This kind of coverage has conditioned Americans to accept autism as the mysterious condition that experts just can't figure out but that they're not really worried about, either.

Meanwhile the autism generation is aging into adulthood with nowhere to go. This is the real autism disaster. This will be the final proof that autism is an epidemic of recent origin.

We've never had a significant adult population like this, and we're doing nothing to prepare for them. Epidemics have come and gone in human history, but the victims either recovered or died. They didn't live long lives dependent on the rest of the population for their support and care, which is what the victims of autism are going to do. And when that happens, the American people will want to know why no one warned them this was coming. Why didn't officials do everything to address autism as a health care emergency? Why didn't doctors sound an alarm over all the sick kids that weren't here twenty years ago? And why didn't the press honestly and thoroughly report on what autism was doing to our children?

People trust that health officials are doing everything they can about autism—they're looking for answers and telling us everything they know. And people believe that members of the media are doing their jobs. If there were really something going on here, reporters would be talking about it. That's the way the system is supposed to work.

# CHAPTER ONE
# UNANSWERED QUESTIONS

*"The release of the paper was greeted with media silence. I spoke to journalists who flat out told me that their networks or their editors were pressured to not cover this story. One highly placed investigative journalist at a major network told me, 'I can't believe what you found. This should be our lead story. It's shocking. And I've been told that I can't cover it.'"*

—Louis Conte on the media's failure to cover "Unanswered Questions."

May 10, 2011, was an important date in the ongoing controversy over vaccines and autism in the US. That was when the report "Unanswered Questions from the Vaccine Injury Compensation Program: A Review of Compensated Cases of Vaccine-Induced Brain Injury" was published in the Pace University *Environmental Law Review*.[1] This report was the culmination of a two-year investigation into the records of the US Vaccine Injury Compensation Program (VICP). There were four authors of the paper: Mary Holland, a law professor at NYU, Louis Conte, a probation officer in Westchester County, NY, and Robert Krakow and Lisa Colin, both attorneys who handle vaccine injury cases in the program.

These four people have something else in common. They are parents of children with autism. Their report in the *Environmental Law Review* was the result of months of work by a number of people sifting through the often incomplete and confusing records of the VICP. The authors put together the individual cases of children injured by vaccines, and they came up with the stunning results showing that in eighty-three cases, the federal government had compensated families where the child became autistic following routine vaccination. All together, they had examined about 200 of the official cases heard by the federal government.

Despite the obscurity of the program, this announcement should have sent shock waves through official agencies. Lawmakers should have taken notice. Most important of all, the national media should have been asking lots of questions.

For years, doctors, health officials, and news outlets had unfailingly denied a link between vaccines and autism. They told the public that lots of studies had been done and there was no evidence that vaccines had anything to do with a child developing autism.

So why had the federal government compensated these children? Why hadn't anyone brought this to light before? Some of these cases went back more than twenty years. What was really going on here? How many more cases like these were yet undiscovered?

"Unanswered Questions" had an important opening question: "Is the Vaccine Injury Compensation Program ('VICP') of the US Court of Federal Claims a fair forum?" Considering how this program is set up and how it functions, the answer in the minds of many would have to be "No." First of all, parents dutifully taking their children in for routine vaccinations are most likely unaware of existence of the VICP. They're also probably not informed that if their child is injured by a vaccine, neither the doctor nor the vaccine maker has any liability.

The *Law Review* article stated, "Under the 1986 National Childhood Vaccine Injury Act ("1986 Law"), Congress created an administrative forum that it meant to ensure simple justice for children; it gave the VICP original jurisdiction for all vaccine injury claims." This empowered the federal government to decide if a vaccine injury claim was valid and should be compensated. In reality, it put parents of vaccine-injured children up against government lawyers defending a government program, using government money.

The issue became more complicated because the question now being asked by more and more concerned parents was: Can vaccines cause a child to become autistic? The official denials had been out there for years. Experts at the Centers for Disease Control and Prevention announced successive studies, all showing no association. How then could it be that the federal government continued to deny a link while recognizing individual cases of vaccine-induced autism?

The study covered in the *Pace Environmental Law Review* revealed that within the 2,500 claims of vaccine injury that have been compensated by the Court of Federal Claims since 1986, eighty-three were found to involve children who became autistic as a result of their vaccinations. Since the creation of the VICP, the government had adamantly denied ever compensating a child for vaccine-induced autism.

By 2005, there were almost five thousand claims filed by parents that vaccines had caused their child to develop autism. The implications here were massive. Eventually, the VICP came up with several autism-vaccine test cases in which the decision reached would then apply to all the other claims. These four cases were known as the Omnibus Autism Proceeding, and the final judgments would directly affect the five thousand claims of a causal link between vaccines and autism waiting to be heard in federal vaccine court.

While the Omnibus Autism Proceeding would set the precedent for denying the existing claims that "autism" could result from vaccinations, the government had long been compensating children who suffered "encephalopathy" (altered brain function) and "residual seizure disorder" because of the vaccines they received. Officials now needed to answer the question: Are there differences in the symptoms exhibited by children with encephalopathy and those labeled autistic? Is this just splitting a very fine hair over the terms used to describe the same condition?

"Unanswered Questions" pointed out that the definition of "autistic disorder" in the official *Diagnostic and Statistical Manual for Mental Disorders* is similar to "the VICP's definitions of 'encephalopathy, seizures and sequela.'"

The Pace article went into detail on how the Vaccine Injury Compensation Program works. The VICP, as it was set up by Congress, was supposed to be a "no fault program under which awards could be made to vaccine-injured persons quickly, easily, and with certainty and generosity."

Back in 1986, parents of vaccine-injured children first had to file a claim with the VICP, which was under the control of the Court of Federal Claims in Washington, D.C. If the case failed to be heard or lost in federal court, parents could still pursue a claim in state courts. This whole thing hinged on the belief that there were "relatively few who were injured by vaccines." As it turned out, this was not really the case.

Despite the pretense that the government had set up a generous program to provide for children whose "futures have been destroyed" and who face "mounting expenses," the conditions that had to be met and the limited table of acceptable vaccine injuries meant few children could actually qualify to file a claim.

As "Unanswered Questions" revealed, "All the injuries on the Vaccine Injury Table were to have occurred within thirty days of vaccination. Most injuries listed on the Table described events that must occur within hours or three days of a child receiving a vaccine."

The relatively few parents with a recognized claim in federal vaccine court, as it came to be called, found themselves opposed by the US Department of Health and Human Services and the Justice Department, not the manufacturer of the vaccine that injured their child. The fact that the vaccine makers themselves had absolutely no liability in federal court meant this industry had been given a unique disincentive to produce a truly safe product.

Instead of having their case heard in a real courtroom with a judge and jury, claimants in the VICP have their petitions heard by one of eight "special masters" from the Court of Federal of Claims. Incredibly, "decisions of the special masters do not serve as precedent in subsequent proceedings in state or federal court." The fact that one child's vaccine injury was recognized had nothing to with the next case where a child experienced that exact same situation of vaccine damage.

In order to address the mounting backlog of 5,000 cases involving autism as a vaccine injury, the VICP would use the test-case decision of parents alleging that the live virus mumps-measles-rubella vaccine caused autism and the test-case decision of parents alleging that the mercury-based vaccine preservative thimerosal caused autism to thimerosal, caused autism, to apply to all the other autism-vaccine claims.

In 2009, three test cases involving the MMR, Michelle Cedillo, Colten Snyder, and Yates Hazlehurst, failed in federal court. That meant that all the claims of autism resulting from this vaccine were denied. The same thing happened with the cases involving thimerosal. Two of the decisions were appealed, but they also failed in the Federal Court of Appeals, and, by 2010, all 5,000 petitioners were informed that their cases had been dismissed.

The judicial double standard was undeniable and deeply troubling to parents with autistic children. Despite the fact that thousands of vaccine-autism cases were now thrown out by the VICP, dozens of others making the same claims had been routinely compensated. "Unanswered Questions" contained a table of twenty-one of the compensated cases listing the case name and the description of the symptoms of autism or autism-like behavior.

> [H]er behavior, which includes head banging, pulling her own hair, and scratching at things, must be constantly redirected. Her disruptive and non-compliant behavior has become a major barrier to progress in functioning.
>
> His mental development has been arrested. . . . He doesn't speak and will never communicate verbally. He doesn't respond to verbal communication. He is not toilet trained. . . . He is self-destructive and very difficult to manage. He needs constant one-on-one care to protect him from injuring himself and others.
>
> Jennifer is a severely mentally retarded individual with hyperactive and destructive behaviors. . . . Her social functioning is extremely inappropriate and she is belligerent and sometimes aggressive. . . . She practices self-stimulating behaviors and she repeatedly bites her hand. She presents a danger to herself and to family members.
>
> Richelle's disabilities include autistic-like behavior, hyperactivity, and partially controlled seizures.
>
> Respondent argues that Eric's current behavior manifestations and retardation fit the pattern of autistic spectrum disorders . . .
>
> They further allege Sarah developed autism and behavior problems as the sequelae of her Table injury.
>
> Seventeen of these twenty-one cases . . . mention the word "autism" or "autistic" or one of the autistic disorders. . . .

"Unanswered Questions" also described in detail how investigators uncovered the cases where the federal government compensated children for vaccine injuries that may have included autism. Volunteers phoned these families and asked specific questions about their child's vaccine injury and about their experience with the VICP. These were not leading questions. A number of the families that reported behaviors associated with autism were then looked at more extensively. A questionnaire was designed by three physicians according to the criteria used by professionals to diagnose autism, and it was used to determine if a child really had symptoms of autism.

After finding these eighty-three compensated cases, the authors of "Unanswered Questions" called for more investigation by the government.

"This discussion must start with the caveat that we are able to only interpret the subgroup of eighty-three compensated cases that we have located. Out of a total number of approximately 2,500 compensated vaccine injury claims, we recognize that this is a small subset. It is our hope that this preliminary study will lead to a more complete study of all cases of compensated vaccine injury. Such a study might provide a far more comprehensive understanding of vaccine injury.

"Despite its limitations, this study suggests that compensated cases of vaccine-induced encephalopathy associated with autism started with the inception of the VICP in 1989 and have continued at least through 2010. Of these eighty-three compensated cases including autism, seventeen note an autistic disorder in a published decision of the Court of Federal Claims, and twenty-two have SCQ questionnaires confirming caregiver reports of autism. In other words, thirty-nine of the eighty-three cases, or 47 percent of this sample, have confirmation of autism beyond parental report alone. The evidence of an association in these cases between recognized vaccine injuries (encephalopathy and residual seizure disorders) and autism exists."

"Unanswered Questions" reported on the fact that the government has never acknowledged what was going on under the supervision of the Department of Health and Human Services and the Department of Justice. The Court of Federal Claims may have been paying out millions for vaccine damages that included autism, but, officially, they said nothing about it.

> It is notable that over a twenty year period the VICP did not publicly acknowledge an apparent vaccine-encephalopathy-autism link. While in the early years of the program there might have been no particular attention to this association, certainly by the late 1990s, the question of vaccine injury and autism was one of general public interest. The finding of so many cases of autism among compensated cases calls into question HHS's assertions on the topic.
>
> Several of the damage awards that HHS compensated included expenses uniquely related to autism. For example, such expenses included Applied Behavioral Analysis ("ABA"), a form of instructional intervention created and used for individuals on the autism spectrum. In other cases, VICP-appointed life planners recommended that families install a fence as the child would be likely to wander later in life. Wandering is a well-recognized characteristic and danger for children with autism. . . .
>
> The authors also received medical and educational records confirming the children's autism diagnoses for some of the compensated cases.

"Unanswered Questions" also described what happened to individual children and what their lives are like today.

> A. is profoundly autistic. She is non-verbal, has major behavioral issues, is self-injurious . . . classic and very severe autism. . . . She cannot be left alone ever. . . . A. was a beautiful baby, who was developing normally, but who had obvious reactions to her first two DPT vaccines. One left her leg swollen and red, and she developed a high fever and screamed after the other. But the doctors did not hesitate to give A. her third DPT shot when she was five months old, and she went over the edge. She had the shot at 4:00 p.m., and by 6:00 p.m. she had a fever of 105 degrees. . . . After that day, she was gone.
>
> B. (aged 44) has no speech, no functional use of his hands, and will no longer stand. . . . He has a couple of seizures every day. . . . B's teeth had to be pulled out because he would not allow anyone near his mouth to brush them. He is not potty trained. He is very sensory defensive, flaps his hands, and makes moaning noises.
>
> C. is a 'giant baby' because although she is an overweight eighteen-year-old, she functions at the level of a two-year-old. She has no life really, compared to her peers. She has very little functional communication and can only say a few words, like "eat" or short phrases that she repeats incessantly . . . She is still in diapers, with no probability that she will ever be potty trained. . . . C. now has frequent periods (every four to six months) of frustration, extreme rage, and self-injurious behavior.

It was also noted in "Unanswered Questions" that even though these parents had vaccine injury claims that were recognized and compensated by the federal government, they were not satisfied with how they were treated.

When parents were asked the simple question, "Was your child's claim resolved fairly?" they responded,

> No, it was a war.
>
> DOJ attorneys were disrespectful and combative. . . . The compensation program should be about compensation and not about defense of the vaccine program.
>
> The attorney for the government was absolutely horrible. She was cold, insulting, and did whatever she could to keep us from being compensated. She pushed for C. to be put in a group home because it would be cheaper than allowing her to live with her family, and she argued against very basic home safety devices like latches on cupboards, a fence for the yard, and a special swing where C. would not fall out when a seizure hit.

These parents saw the need for serious changes in the way the compensation program works.

> The court spends far too much time looking for ways *not* to compensate families.
>
> It should be overhauled.
>
> There should be a program in place that would allow the court to reassess children later in life to see if their needs have changed. This would make the life care planning less contentious and would allow for changes in laws, insurance coverage, and mostly the child's level of functioning. It is ridiculous to assume that you can adequately plan when a child is very young for every possible consequence of the vaccine damage throughout the child's life.

The Pace report pointed out the sobering truth that while a parent expects the government to do something for a child harmed by a vaccine, the program is set up to insure that as few injuries as possible are recognized.

> "The overwhelming majority of petitioners in the VICP have not received compensation. Of the 13,755 claims filed in the VICP to date, 2,621 awards have been paid, or less than one in five of total number of claims filed. So far, 5,277 claims have been dismissed and 5,857 claims are pending. As most of the pending cases are in the Omnibus, they are likely to be dismissed. The March 3, 2011, HHS Statistics Report notes that 'HHS has never concluded in any case that autism was caused by vaccination.'"

One important unanswered question was how many more cases of autism are among the several thousand children compensated for vaccine damage. Is the government at all curious? Does anyone hold officials accountable to find out?

The report asked,

> (1) Were HHS and DOJ aware of the prevalence of autism diagnoses among those who have been compensated for encephalopathy and residual seizure disorder?
>
> (2) What percentage of the remaining VICP-compensated cases of vaccine-induced injuries manifest autism?
>
> (3) Is "autism" perhaps a different term for slightly less severe encephalopathy and residual seizure disorder? Is it possible that 'autism' is a form of brain damage similar to acute encephalopathy and residual seizure disorder but vaccine-induced brain damage all the same? This argument has been made for over two decades; unfortunately, the hypothesis has been inadequately studied.

"Unanswered Questions" also wanted to know if the real problem here is the use of the word "autism."

> Some may argue that vaccines indirectly caused autism as a result of other vaccine-induced brain damage. Whether autism is considered a secondary injury to encephalopathy and residual seizure disorder or a primary injury appears to be a semantic point having little legal significance. Under either theory, vaccines led to brain injury, and the VICP has compensated that vaccine-induced brain injury, including autism. In other words, HHS has been compensating certain expenses of vaccine-induced autism for more than twenty years when labeled as "encephalopathy" and "residual seizure disorder" but not compensating it when labeled "autism" without cogent explanation.

What is the truth here? Can it be that the government does, on occasion, agree with overwhelming evidence that yes, vaccines do cause autism? Do they do it in such a manner that the public never hears about it? Is that the reason that they can still maintain that vaccines are never the direct cause of autism?

The authors of "Unanswered Questions" called on Congress to look into this. This seemingly double standard regarding autism and vaccines cannot continue. Either autism is a side effect of vaccination or it isn't. They cannot have it both ways.

> Autism is the most prevalent developmental disorder in the United States . . . This preliminary evaluation suggests that vaccine-induced encephalopathy and seizure disorder may be associated with autism. We recommend that Congress open an investigation of all compensated cases of vaccine-induced injury to find out how frequently this association occurs. Congress should find out what HHS, DOJ, and the VICP knew about the existence of autism as a characteristic of those compensated for encephalopathy and residual seizure disorder.

"Unanswered Questions" concluded by saying,

> While there are likely many routes to "autism," including neurological insults and toxic post-natal exposures, this preliminary analysis of VICP-compensated cases suggests that autism is also associated with vaccine-induced brain damage. . . .
>
> Based on this preliminary assessment, there may be no meaningful distinction between cases of encephalopathy and residual seizure disorder that the VICP compensated over the last twenty years and the cases of "autism" that the VICP has denied. If true, this would be a profound injustice to those denied recovery and to all those who have invested trust in this system that Congress created. This preliminary study calls for Congress to investigate the VICP and for scientists to investigate all compensated cases of vaccine injury to gain a fuller understanding of the totality of consequences of vaccine injury.

Parents and advocates had to act quickly when "Unanswered Questions" was published. They had to make sure this information reached more people than just the readers of the *Pace University Environmental Law Review.*

Actually the day before, on May 9, 2011, in a Fox News exclusive called *Government Paid Millions to Vaccine-Injured Kids,* reporter Alisyn Camerota publicized the "groundbreaking announcement" that would take place on May 10 in Washington D.C.[2] She did this in an interview with one of the mothers involved in the study, a psychologist, Dr. Sarah Bridges. Camerota began by saying that there would be a major announcement shortly. An investigation had found dozens of families with vaccine-injured children who had been compensated by the federal government. These injuries included autism. Dr. Bridges was one of these parents. Camerota asked her why she believed that her son's autism was the result of the vaccines he had received. Sarah Bridges said that the evidence was overwhelming. He was a normal, healthy baby until his check-up at four months. He got a number of shots at that doctor visit, and the reaction was immediate. That very night he was sick. He woke his parents with a high-pitched scream and become unconscious. His temperature was 106. He began seizing. Doctors had to sedate him to the point of not breathing in order to stop the seizures. From that point on, according to Dr. Bridges, all his disabilities began—including his descent into autism.

Camerota brought up the government's double speak, namely that while officials continue to say there is no link between vaccines and autism, these cases show that they do recognize a link. Parents have received compensation. She also mentioned the case of Hannah Poling, whose claim of vaccine induced autism was conceded by medical experts at HHS, although it was alleged to be so unique because of her underlying mitochondrial condition that there were probably no other cases like hers. Camerota asked Bridges how much she received from the government.

Bridges said that her son had been awarded millions by the US government for what vaccines did to him—mental retardation, seizures, autism—but there were a number of strings attached. Every penny must be accounted for, right down to the cost of the diapers. She said it is paid out in an annual annuity, and, when they were figuring these costs, she was told things like, "A lot of kids don't live to be very old with this disability"

Camerota pointed up the contradiction involved in this. The government has never publicly admitted a link between vaccines and autism. They've always cited the studies showing that there was no connection, but this news, "in some ways, smacks of a cover-up." She then asked Bridges if she was ever told to keep quiet about the settlement. Bridges answered, "Very routinely."

She said that she was told that this is an annuity. It could be stopped. She was warned not to talk about it. Because of all the secrecy surrounding her settlement, she admitted that she had "no idea how prevalent this was."

Bridges went on to describe the toll autism had taken on her family. Her marriage ended. Her other children were severely impacted, and her disabled son ended up being placed in a home because of his critical needs.

Camerota continued saying that the next day, May 10, 2011, dozen of families would be "taking the bold step" of making an announcement in Washington. This would be done despite the fact that families had been told "to be quiet because the money could dry up for care."

Bridges talked about that announcement. She said it was "a red herring" for the government to claim that there was no link between vaccines and autism. Her child had been compensated in 2001. Dozens of other children also had their claims recognized by the government. Even one exception meant that the government's claim was invalid. She added that there was a risk in parents doing this. Some parents were not willing to do this. Bridges felt that she was one of the "lucky ones" and therefore she felt "a real obligation to do that."

Camerota pointed out that these parents are not anti-vaccine. They simply want the risks publicized.

Bridges agreed. She said that there's probably a genetic susceptibility that puts "a very few number of people" at risk. She stated that she was "very pro-vaccine" and there were some that would be injured for "the public good." Her concern was the government's reluctance to recognize and care for the children who were injured. "To me, that is completely immoral. That's where the victimization happened to me, not in the fact that we were unfortunate to be one of the few that was injured."

Fox News then included an expert to present the other side.

Camerota said that what Sarah Bridges presented was "tough evidence to refute," Dr. Cynara Comer, assistant professor of surgery at Mount Sinai Medical Center, responded.

Comer said that parents weren't actually being compensated for autism, but for brain damage, at the same time she said, "Autism apparently seems to be one of the illnesses that they were awarding money for." She cautioned that "we have to be very, very careful about this." She said she was very sympathetic for Dr. Bridges because her son was "quote, unquote, and I don't mean this in a bad way, damaged, or hurt, by these vaccinations, or injured by these vaccinations."

Comer cited the studies that show vaccines are safe and beneficial and that these benefits outweighed the risks. "And although autism has been implicated as causing injuries from vaccinations, or being . . . as autism has been, implicated in vaccinations, we have to also look at the other studies that have shown that autism . . has not been caused by vaccinations."

Camerota then brought up the distinction between the use of the term "encephalopathy" and the term "autism" with Dr. Bridges. Bridges said that "encephalopathy" is the medical term for "brain injury." The government may use the word "encephalopathy" in acknowledging a vaccine injury that resulted in autism, but according to her, "this is real word play." She said, "The real crime is when we then have children who are damaged for the public good, that we don't take care of properly."

It was encouraging for parents to see Fox News cover this so thoroughly. Many thought that what was happening might finally force the government, mainstream medicine, and the rest of the media to honestly address this controversy.

Fox News continued their extraordinary coverage of this critical event on May 10, 2011, in a report called *Law School Links Autism, Vaccines in Report.* Camerota began the interview by that saying that regardless of all the official statements, "the feds have been quietly compensating children injured by vaccines. These are children who have autism, all this, despite the public denials." Camerota asked Holland why this announcement was so important.

Holland pointed out the obvious contradiction. The government says that they have never recognized a link between vaccines and autism, yet here are dozens of cases. She called for answers. "We want Congress to hold hearings."[3]

Camerota acknowleged that the authors of the study are "not disinterested" since all of them have autistic children. Two of them are lawyers who've represented vaccine-injured children. She asked about the objectivity of the findings.

According to Holland, the facts speak for themselves. They found eighty-three cases exploring the government's data. She said that these cases can be verified by the Department of Justice and by Health and Human Services. These were the facts. Holland explained, "I think the fact that we are stakeholders in this issue goes to our motivation. I don't think it goes to bias."

Asked about the amounts of the settlements, Holland said the anounts varied. Some of the annuities involved tens of thousands of dollars and some amounted to millions. "We're talking about really large sums of money with these families who have children who are severely injured by vaccines and they also have autism."

Camerota brought up what Dr. Bridges had said about the secret nature of these settlements. Bridges had been told not to talk about it. Camerota said it was implied that going public could put her annuity at risk. What had other families been told? Holland couldn't speak for the families who'd been compensated in that regard, but the information about the settlements was found in federal docket reports and published judicial decisions. This was indisputable.

The discussion then turned to the repercussions from this news. Camerota noted that millions of children get vaccinated and have no problem. She asked if talking about eighty-three cases of vaccines and autism might create "a public panic." What if parents stopped vaccinating because of it?

Mary Holland said, "We're not anti-vaccine, but we are anti-vaccine injury. I think we can all agree that children should get the safest vaccines humanly possible, and that those children who have the grave misfortune to be injured by their childhood vaccines should be compensated." She emphasized that we have to create a fair and just compensation program. The public should be told the truth about vaccine injury.

Government officials had been asked for a response to this announcement, and Camerota read a statement saying that the government had found no link between the MMR vaccine and autism. Holland was asked for her reaction to the government's position.

Mary Holland noted that there were epidemiological studies backing what the government said, but she reminded everyone that the cases that had been compensated were also based on scientific evidence. Holland said that decisions often rested on the use of the word "autism," regardless of the fact that the injuries are almost identical. She again called for Congress to investigate this federal program.,

Fox then had their legal analyst, Mercedes Colwin, comment about these eighty-three compensated cases. Camerota asked what it would mean if every case of a child who developed autism after being vaccinated had to be compensated by the government.

Colwin called it a "colossal slippery slope argument" because the implications were enormous. She made a reference to Hannah Poling, the nine-year-old who "got compensated with millions of dollars" and the possibility that there would be "frivolous claims." The cost of an onslaught of vaccine injury cases seemed to be more of a concern to Colwin than the fact that the government had secretly recognized autism as a vaccine injury while denying it publicly. "If they're victorious, we're talking about millions and millions of dollars in recovery for each child."

Next, Camerota asked Mary Holland what the eighty-three cases would mean for the thousands of cases awaiting a decision in "vaccine court."

Although Holland didn't think it would affect the cases directly, she hoped it would cause people to ask their representatives in Washington to take action. Since the vaccine program affected every child, the compensation program should be a concern for every parent.

With this kind of initial media coverage, one would expect that there would be lots of follow-up by various print and TV news outlets. They would have no choice but to cover the announcement of the VICP study. How could they not talk about it? This was the most heated controversy in pediatric medicine. If all these kids with autism had been compensated for vaccine injury by the government, it was a direct contradiction of everything ever said by US health officials.

Those listening to what the speakers said on May 10, 2011, in front of the Court of Federal Claims in Washington, understood that these were serious charges being made.[4]

Mary Holland, Louis Conte, Dr. Sarah Bridges, Bob Krakow, and Lisa Colin spoke.

Mary Holland began her remarks saying that their study had just been published in an article called "Unanswered Questions," in the *Pace Environmental Law Review*, a peer-reviewed journal. She went on to say that despite the official denials from both the Vaccine Injury Compensation Program and the Department of Health and Human Services, dozens of children compensated for vaccine injuries have autism. Holland quoted the HHS website saying, "[HHS] has never concluded in any case that autism was caused by vaccination," and that furthermore, in 2010, the

Omnibus Autism Proceeding, the Court of Federal Claims and the Federal Circuit Court of Appeal had both rejected claims that vaccines cause autism. But, Holland pointed out the reality that "it is widely medically accepted that vaccines can cause brain damage and injury. They can even cause death. But HHS and the Vaccine Injury Compensation Program have made clear that they've concluded that vaccines do not cause autism."

Given their strong position denying any connection between the vaccine program and autism, Holland said that one would expect that no vaccine injury case would involve autism. But, she said, "that's not what we found in our preliminary study . . . based only on the government's own records." "Unanswered Questions" revealed that there were twenty-one cases "that associate vaccine injury and autism." In addition, there were "sixty-two settlement agreements where HHS paid damages, without trial, to victims of vaccine injury who have autism. We found eighty-three cases in all of autism associated with vaccine injury. And we think this is the tip of the iceberg."

Holland described how these children were assessed in order to confirm that they actually had autism. "There was confirmation beyond parental report." In one startling statement, she said, "Based on their eighty-three cases, the autism prevalence rate among those vaccine-injured is at least three times higher than among US children today."

Holland brought up the puzzling double standard on the part of those deciding who gets compensated. "Our study suggests that the program has compensated many cases of vaccine injury associated with autism when the word is not used, and has rejected claims of vaccine injury when the word 'autism' is used."

Next Louis Conte talked about how the investigation was conducted. He said that ten trained volunteers "gathered [the] information that was synthesized in this article." And for him, it was personal, too. Two of his triplet boys have autism.

Conte cited the case of Hannah Poling, the Georgia girl whose injury claim was conceded by the federal government in 2008. Hannah Poling has autism. She was a healthy child who suddenly and dramatically regressed into autism following routine vaccinations. Medical experts at HHS agreed, and she was awarded millions in compensation. Conte noted that the government said she suffers from "autism-like symptoms" as a result of her vaccinations, along with brain damage and seizures. The Poling case failed to set any precedents and was declared to be "a rare, freak occurrence."

The authors of "Unanswered Questions" didn't accept that what happened to Hannah Poling was so uncommon. They asked themselves how many other cases of vaccine-induced autism had been quietly settled by the federal government without going to vaccine court. Conte said that with assistance from Pace Law School, they had spent two years investigating vaccine settlements and claims of autism. They sifted through records, interviewed families, and compiled the data that was published in the article. Based on what they found, Conte said, "We suspect that there are many more compensated cases that we did not find."

Next, parents spoke about what vaccine injuries were like for their children. Dr. Sarah Bridges, a psychologist from Minneapolis who had been interviewed the previous day on Fox News, spoke first. Her son was damaged by his vaccines. The government agreed, and he received compensation. All the experts who deal with her son, his doctors, his teachers, his therapists, say he has autism, according to his mother. So why is it that the government continues to say that "vaccines never have a linkage to autism"? Bridges wanted to know. "My son was compensated ten years ago, and the government continues to pay for all of his autism treatments. The formal diagnosis of my son, Porter, is brain injury. He has a brain injury that's led to mental retardation, seizures, and autism. He's also hyperactive. He requires twenty-four hour care."

Dr. Bridges went to say that her son is one of four children and had been born "perfectly healthy" in 1993. It was when he was four months old, at his well-baby checkup, that everything changed. He dramatically reacted to the vaccinations, and, as his mother attested, "That started an odyssey of hospitalizations, of doctors, of medications, of therapies, that culminated in Porter having a case in the vaccine court." Bridges acknowledged that they were one of the rare cases to have a win in "vaccine court." The victory is nothing to celebrate, however. She said, "I have a seventeen-year-old boy who wears a helmet and has diapers on. My marriage crumbled during this. The other kids fell apart. The stress was unbelievable, culminating in my son being placed in a home so that he could get round-the-clock care."

Then Sue Leteure of Centerville, Tennessee, spoke. She came forward with her daughter Kimberly. Kimberly was clearly disabled. She didn't seem to have any awareness of her surroundings. At the same time her mother spoke, she held on to her daughter with both of her hands to keep her from walking away. Louis Conte came over and assisted Sue Leteure with her daughter so she could make her remarks. Leteure described what had happened. "Kimberly is a vaccine injury child. She was nine weeks old when she had her initial shot. We are very blessed to have her as good as she is. She has mental retardation. She has seizures. She has autistic tendencies, and a lot of autism showed up when she was probably eighteen months old. She has had thousands of seizures over the years. We also were able to win a suit for her."

As she stood, trying to control her daughter, she said simply, "Money doesn't compensate for loss of life."

Despite the charge that's often made against anyone who talks about vaccine side effects, Sue Leteure stated adamantly, "As with most of our parents, I'm not anti-vaccine. We need a safer vaccine for our children. We need to be able to protect them." She struggled with the words, "If the government is aware of what's happening, we need to have the support from all of them to take care of our children, to immunize safely, and to make sure that the autism in this community stops."

Finally, she pointed out the frightening situation most parents of autistic children face. "Where we were able to win our compensation for Kimberly, I know that as a parent, my daughter will be taken care of when she is older. We were initially one of the first ones because this happened in 1981 . . . And we want to stop this from happening to anyone else."

Leteure ended by saying that her daughter had been a normal child up until her nine-month doctor's visit. Suddenly she got sick and was brain injured, resulting in seizures and autism. Again she asked for safer vaccines and just compensation for injured children. "Later in life, who's going to take care of them? They deserve better."

More parents then addressed the press conference. Ed and Joyce Alger of Palm Bay, Florida, were next, talking about their son, Danny. Ed held up a photo of his son and showed it slowly to those in attendance. He said that he could "only echo the statements of the previous speakers." He, too, could recount endless stories about seizures, injuries, and hospital visits. Instead, he said, "Our Danny Louis . . . was born a perfect baby. . . . He was a loving, bubbling, babbling, beautiful baby boy. And we only got to enjoy that for four months."

It was at four months that they lost their beautiful baby. Danny's dad recounted that the same day that he was vaccinated, he let out "a terrible scream." Those who heard the scream thought that "a wild animal had gotten in the house in the basement." His son became inconsolable, constantly screaming and his body becoming stiff. They were told that Danny was having seizures. He didn't make eye contact and was constantly in motion, according to his father. "He enjoyed waving his hands in front of his face for no apparent reason." The father now knows these were signs of autism.

Alger described the severity of Danny's injuries. "Right now, as a result . . . from the initial shot, another injustice, Danny is also paralyzed on the right side. He's confined to a hospital bed. He's on every medicine you can imagine, but he continues to seizure." Ed said Danny having seizures is "the norm."

Again, here were parents who still support the vaccine program. "We believe vaccines are not always safe for everybody . . . and we believe they can cause autism. Our son Daniel is proof."

Incredibly, this happened to the Alger family thirty years ago. Ed said that parents today are still being told vaccines don't cause autism. "We proved them wrong then, and I think we can prove them wrong now." He ended by asking for Congress do something.

(On Tuesday, April 29, 2014, Danny Alger, age thirty-seven, died from complications resulting from his vaccine injury.)

The next speaker, Debbie Fields, was also from Minneapolis. She described her son Andrew and his vaccine injury at fifteen months of age. Despite having an ear infection, he was given four shots. In the days that followed, he began to change, and, by day ten, he had a seizure in his mother's arms. He began losing words, and and his temperament changed. He became hyperactive. By age three, he was diagnosed with autism. Today, Andrew is eighteen years old. Debbie said, "Andrew received compensation from the Vaccine Injury Compensation Program for the MMR that [he] was given that day. The government, medicine, and the media contend that vaccines have never caused autism. Look at the case of my son, and and you decide if the government has really told the truth."

When Bob Krakow had his turn to speak, his words were powerful. "Alger, Bridges, Fields, Leteure, seventy-nine more that we found, and we're still counting. They say it is impossible that vaccines would be associated with autism. We're finding that the impossible has already happened, and that's why we're here today. We want to send a message and show the nation the window that we've opened to the truth. . . . We need justice, just simple justice for our children."

Krakow also said Congress should hold hearings and get this out in the open. The system that Congress set up in 1986 was intended to give immunity to the pharmaceutical industry and provide fair treatment of those who were injured by vaccines. Bob said only the first part of that has been realized.

Finally, Mary Holland called on Congress to find out how this association could be "hidden in plain sight." She asked a simple question: "Is this program fulfilling the job Congress set for it?" And she also said that we need Congress "to commission an independent medical inquiry into all the cases of compensated vaccine injury so that we can better understand the totality of consequences of vaccine injury."

During the questions that followed, the individual parents again affirmed the fact that they weren't advising the public not to vaccinate. Sarah Bridges added the troubling comment that "in ten years, no one has ever, ever followed up with our family about . . . 'How is your child doing?' 'He was brain injured by a vaccine.' Or, 'Wow, your child has autism and was compensated. Maybe we should look at these children and figure out what is special about your kid. Can we learn something about genetics?' That kind of research, that kind of exploration is not going on. And frankly, I find it completely unacceptable and immoral."

And on May 11, the day after the press conference at the Court of Federal Claims, Fox News in Boston reported that the federal government had been compensating vaccine-injured children who had autism in an interview with the mother of a vaccine-injured son with autism, Heather McLennand, and Northwest University pharmacology professor Dr. Richard Deth.[5]

Fox 25 Boston announced that even though many thought the idea of a link between vaccines and autism "had been put to rest," parents were presenting the research that "again points to vaccine as the cause."

McLennand started off talking about her son, Liam, who was born November 11, 2003. She said he was a typical healthy baby until he went to his three-month doctor visit, where he got three vaccines. By that evening, he was screaming uncontrollably. The following day, his mother found blood in his stool. McLennand said that she later learned that this is a sign of a vaccine injury. The next day, his doctor said he seemed okay.

McLennand said she continued to have her son vaccinated. Each time, he had a reaction, but then he seemed to recover. Finally after his eighteen-month vaccines, "his health just went crazy." Just before he turned four, he was diagnosed with autism.

The news anchor addressed Dr. Deth about the eighty-three cases. Did he believe that these compensated cases showed that vaccines and autism are linked?

Deth said, "I very much agree with that." He cited the studies that show vaccination can cause inflammation and oxidative damage that can lead to autism and other neurodevelopmental problems.

Deth then explained how the inflammation caused by vaccination could lead to autism. He made a case for how the vaccine response can cause neuro-inflammation and systemic inflammation in kids with autism. He said that tests of these children showed that they have this inflammation as a result of being vaccinated.

The discussion turned to the question of it being just a coincidence that kids show signs of autism when they've been vaccinated. Deth said that some kids show abnormal signs from the time they're born, but more and more children are just fine until they're vaccinated. Then they change, stop talking, lose skills, and end up with autism. This happening at the time they're vaccinated is a clear sign of a temporal relationship, according to Deth.

The news anchor asked about the position of officials from the Centers for Disease Control and Prevention who have said there is no link. "Is this a cover-up, in your opinion?"

Deth responded that the CDC's goal is to promote vaccines.

> That's their agenda. They conduct epidemiological or large-population studies, but they don't do research looking at individual children.

Deth said that the CDC was "missing the boat when it comes to . . . what really causes autism on the individual child level."

Fox 25 wanted to know what this might do to parents' attitudes about vaccinating, considering that the eighty-three families are "a small percentage of those who have their children vaccinated."

Heather McLennand said this is "a hard question to ask a parent" because she believes "vaccination is incredibly important" despite the fact her child had an adverse reaction to a vaccine. She had her personal criticism of vaccines. She said she thought the vaccine schedule is too big and lacks proper testing. In her child's case, she found he was allergic to some of the ingredients in his vaccines. "He shouldn't have been vaccinated."

Fox 25 asked Dr. Deth about the answer to this dilemma. "[Should] children be tested prior to vaccination?"

Deth said that it would be good to do this, but only if we admit what vaccines are really doing to children. In order for this to happen, the government needs to "come clean on this" and "acknowledge what the risks really are."

Fox was the exception. Where was the *New York Times*, *Washington Post*, ABC, NBC? Wasn't this a major news event? Isn't it the media's job to inform us about government duplicity like this? Why was Fox News the only leading news outlet to give this story the thorough attention that it clearly deserved?

Maybe this revelation was just too stunning, too difficult to explain. After twenty years of these same news sources declaring over and over that all the science is in and nothing connects vaccines to autism, would this be too big a contradiction?

It should be noted that CNN did mention the event in Washington, but they did it in such a way that the real story was neatly covered up.[6] A video showed Mary Holland and the others speaking in front of the Court of Federal Claims with a headline that said, "Possible Autism-Vaccine Link—Group says connection needs a closer look," and a news anchor reported that a "a group of lawyers and families" had just announced that children who received compensation for vaccine injuries "were more likely to be autistic." CNN said the group was urging Congress to look into this "alleged connection." Finally the anchor reminded viewers, "The Centers for Disease Control has long argued against the vaccine-autism link."

Using a voiceover meant no one heard what anyone actually said. Nothing was said about who exactly was speaking or where these people actually were. It sounded like a group of parents and lawyers came to Washington with the tired, old, debunked claim that vaccines cause autism, which CNN was quick to remind us was denied by the CDC.

CNN's coverage was exactly twenty-six seconds.

This was a story that was left to die. This may have been a shocking revelation, but if no one is willing report on it, the public remains ignorant. Mainstream media controls what the American people hear about. In the real world, that's called censorship.

This wasn't the end of the story, however.

During a hearing in the Massachusetts State Assembly in July 2011, a news person made it clear what those who control the media will and will not allow. This hearing was about expanding parental choice in vaccine exemptions, and a number of medical experts and others spoke in favor of the legislation. One of those who addressed lawmakers was Mish Michaels, who had worked in the Boston TV market as a meteorologist for almost twenty years. She said she was also the mother of a four-year-old daughter and a trained scientist and an environment reporter.

Michaels said that her job has been to "ask difficult scientific questions" and go beyond "scientific consensus." She related how she investigated health concerns in 2006, when she became pregnant. Both she and her husband were graduates of Cornell University and had science backgrounds. They studied "what it means to have a healthy child." They were especially concerned because they had a special-needs child in their family. Michaels said this child developed leukemia after "exposure to vaccines and pesticides."

Michaels talked about their "many Ivy League-educated friends" who had children who were autistic. She said she and her husband had many questions. Originally they believed everything they were being told in the news stories about vaccines, but once they started looking into this for themselves, they had "more questions than answers." When they brought their concerns up with their daughter's pediatrician, they "were no longer able to visit the practice." For refusing to vaccinate, they were denied medical care. This caused Mish Michaels to investigate further. She went to the news management at WBZ-TV and showed them the current research she had on vaccines and on vaccine injury. She said, "What I was told time and time again was that there was no story, that the science is settled, that there is no reason to present stories of this nature on TV because simply these are fringe stories."

Michaels found this to be surprising because she thought covering topics like this was the job of media. This affected lots of people, and the media was supposed to be "a voice of the people."

When Michaels discovered the Pace Environmental Law Review stating that there were dozens of children with autism who had been compensated by the US government for vaccine injuries, she was eager to report on it. She and another reporter, Caterina Bandini, tried to interest area stations in the story. For Bandini, this was especially important because one of her twin daughters had autism. Despite their efforts, no news outlet wanted to cover the story. They were told it wasn't worth reporting on because "the science was settled." Fox 25 did cover it, and the response was huge. Michaels said that for five days in a row, it was the number-one news story. She said, "There were hundreds and hundreds of comments from families explaining how their children were vaccine damaged. There were thousands of flags on Facebook."

Then Tuesday, August 23, 2011, HDNet TV World Report broadcast the segment, *Vaccines and Autism: Mixed Signals.*[7] The report was about a half hour in length, and it covered the topic in a thorough and balanced manner. Many parents who were veterans of years of watching media coverage of the vaccine-autism controversy realized that this program was exceptional.

The people included in the story were familiar names to those in the autism community: Michelle Cedillo, Kimberly Sue Leteure, Mary Holland, Becky Estepp, and Louis Conte. The focus was the "Unanswered Questions" piece published three months before that showed that dozens of families who'd been compensated for vaccine injuries have children who have autism.

Louis Conte: "What we did was we looked at the cases of individuals who were compensated for encephalopathy and for seizure disorder, and we asked another question: Does your child also have autism? And in a surprising number of a handful of interviews . . . the answers came back 'Yes.'"

Viewers were told about the similarities between encephalopathy (brain injury) and autism and about the children whose vaccines injuries were compensated and about children with the same injuries who didn't receive compensation. The report revealed the stunning truth that back at the beginning of the government's Vaccine Injury Compensation Program in the 1980s, if a child was injured by vaccines and had symptoms of autism, chances were good that the injury would be recognized as vaccine related. Later in the 1990s, as the number of required vaccines had increased dramatically along with the claims of vaccine damage, the VICP tended to reject the claim.

World Report showed us the personal stories of vaccine injury victims. It was very hard to watch Michelle Cedillo and Kimberly Sue Leteure and ignore the possibility that vaccines are responsible for the severe disabilities both of these girls endured. They were both born healthy and suddenly and dramatically regressed following routine vaccinations. Kimberly Sue won her case in federal court, and Michelle Cedillo lost.

These arbitrary vaccine-injury judgments should have us all concerned. If vaccines aren't responsible for Michelle's disabilities, what is to blame?

"Michelle was one of those test cases. And the government used seventeen expert witnesses to argue against her claim of a vaccine injury, none of them actually having examined her. And in the end, although Kimberly Leteure had won a similar claim a few years earlier, the goalposts seemed to have moved. Michelle, along with each of the other test cases, lost, which basically killed the claims of 5,000 autistic children and every claim since. So if you happened to be born in the 1980s, you were compensated. If you were born after that, you weren't."

Mary Holland said, "I think the key difference between those who are compensated and those who are not is the 'A word.'"

Louis Conte agreed, "If a child from fifteen years ago could get compensated for encephalopathy, but they also had autism, how come a child today who has autism, clearly encephalopathy, and other features as well, just because they have the word 'autism' associated with their case, does that mean they're not to be considered? Or is this really a matter of public policy because we have an increase in autism?"

Becky Estepp's son Eric was featured. He, too, started out as a normal baby boy and was badly impacted repeatedly by his vaccinations, resulting ultimately in autism. And like Michelle Cedillo, he lost in the VICP.

World Report pointed out a number of things that are rarely mentioned in stories about vaccines and autism. Namely, thousands of vaccine-autism claims have been thrown out of the Vaccine Program as a result of the test cases that lost. And what was most revealing in *Mixed Signals* was the absence of any government official who was willing to appear in the story to explain the decisions of the Vaccine Program or to defend the government's position on the vaccine-autism controversy.

"We wanted to interview officials in Washington who would offer the best arguments against the supposition that vaccines can cause autism, but no one would talk. We asked repeatedly to interview someone from the Department of Justice, which argued against the families making claims. Our requests were rejected with the response, 'The court's opinion speaks for itself.'

"We also tried to interview any of the arbitrators from the Vaccine Court, who are called 'special masters,' some of whom had mocked the parents as 'victims of bad science' with 'reconstructed memories' and the doctors who supported them as guilty of 'gross medical misjudgment.' None could do it. We worked with the FDA to get an on-the-record interview. They declined. And we tried repeatedly to interview someone, anyone, from the Department of Health and Human Services, which administers the Vaccine Injury Compensation Fund, including Secretary Kathleen Sebelius. The secretary was quoted last year in *Reader's Digest* saying of those who argue that there's a link between vaccines and autism, 'We have reached out to media outlets to try to get them to not give the views of these people equal weight in their reporting.' When we asked her agency last week whether she had really said that, they responded, 'No one here can remember or determine that this quote is factual.'"

There were legitimate questions raised in this report. This is an issue affecting millions of American families. It is outrageous to learn that no government official was willing to speak publicly and address this controversy.

Even more concerning was this brief comment: "Even a member of the government's Advisory Commission on Childhood Vaccines told us research on vaccine safety remains flawed and incomplete."

Parents have a lot to worry about. If someone working in the vaccine program admits that the science isn't in on vaccine safety, what are we doing to our children?

By a strange coincidence, the leading American autism advocacy group, Autism Speaks, published a surprising announcement at the same time the eighty-three cases were announced.[8] They said that investigators had studied the autism rate in South Korea and had come to the conclusion that the true autism rate there was "2.64%, or approximately one in thirty-eight children, and concluded that autism prevalence estimates worldwide may increase when this approach is used to identify children with ASD." (*AutismSpeaks.org*, May 9, 2011)

Autism Speaks, a group that has endlessly urged us to be aware and "learn the signs," while at the same time financed lots of studies looking for the elusive gene/genes that cause autism, couldn't have timed this better.

If the real rate of autism in South Korea is one in thirty-eight, the same might be true here.

Autism Speaks made it clear that this study wasn't proof that South Korea had more autism than other countries. What this probably showed was the fact that autism was more common than previously thought. If experts really did careful work, they would find the same rate everywhere.

This was related to what had just been announced at the US Court of Federal Claims. Mary Holland had said in her remarks: "Based on their eighty-three cases, the autism-prevalence rate among those vaccine injured is at least three times higher than among US children today."

So, was this timely South Korean study showing an autism rate of one in thirty-eight a convenient way to dismiss the charge that investigators had found significantly more autism among children with a vaccine-injury claim? Autism Speaks had found about three times more autism in South Korean children. So should we expect that it's normal that all these vaccine-injured children would also have autism—a condition that didn't exist until their vaccine injury occurred?

Autism Speaks doesn't speak for parents of children who regressed into autism following routine vaccinations. They're right in line with the official government denial of a causal link. They may hold endless walks to raise money and awareness, but they say very little about why so many children today have autism.

Maybe the real shocking revelation here is that vaccine-injured children are a lot more common than previously thought.

I spoke to Dr. Sarah Bridges two and a half years after the announcement in Washington. The simple fact is that her son was healthy and normal until he was vaccinated. After routine vaccinations, he developed "brain injury, mental retardation, seizures, and autism." Bridges said, "Autism is a result of the brain damage." She has difficulty with the term "autism." "We're really talking about brain injury," she said. Her son received an award totaling seven to eight million dollars for his lifetime care. He gets about a hundred thousand a year to pay for his expenses. She told me that after the 2011 news coverage, "I thought there'd be more interest. I thought people would look at the data."

I also asked one of the authors of "Unanswered Questions," Louis Conte, about what it meant to him after all this was made public.

"Our investigation into the cases compensated for vaccine injury by the federal government through the National Vaccine Injury Compensation Program took over two years. Because the federal government denied our request for access to NVICP information, we spent hundreds of hours reviewing records, locating and interviewing families. This work was done, without pay, in an organized, efficient and—above all—respectful manner.

"We found that the NVICP had compensated eighty-three cases for vaccine-injury-induced brain damage, or encephalopathy, that also featured autism. Given the statements of federal authorities, there shouldn't have been any cases featuring autism. Yet, in getting access to no more than 196 cases (perhaps 15 percent of all of the compensated cases), we found autism to be fairly common.

"This is a significant finding. It shows that autism and encephalopathy are associated. This finding ought to be informing future scientific inquiry. That autism occurred so frequently in cases of vaccine injury ought to have been disclosed. The Department of Health and Human Services knew about the relationship between vaccine-injury-induced encephalopathy and autism and said nothing.

"The release of the paper was greeted with media silence. I spoke to journalists who flat out told me that their networks or their editors were pressured to not cover this story. One highly placed investigative journalist at a major network told me, 'I can't believe what you found. This should be our lead story. It's shocking. And I've been told that I can't cover it.'

"I'm saddened because the public needs to know this information so that they can make informed health care decisions for their children.

"I am also saddened that the families who told us about their vaccine children deserved the respect of a sincere public acknowledgement of their children's suffering.

"It has been over two years since the release of 'Unanswered Questions.' More cases of vaccine-induced brain damage featuring autism have been compensated. The findings have never been acknowledged by the government, nor have they been challenged. The findings stand, defying the silence."

# CHAPTER TWO
# ANDREW WAKEFIELD

*"I'm not here to let you pitch your book. I'm here to have you answer questions."*

—News anchor Anderson Cooper to Dr. Andrew Wakefield on CNN, January 5, 2011

It would be impossible to write a book on how the media covers autism without a chapter on Dr. Andrew Wakefield. His name, more than any other, is tied to the controversial issue of vaccines and autism. To put it simply, the press regularly makes the claim that parents believe vaccines cause autism because of a study by Dr. Wakefield published in the *Lancet*, a British medical journal, back in 1998. The reference is usually very brief, involving only a sentence or two, like in this *Boston Globe* reference from November 2013: "Ever since a British doctor published a study in 1998 suggesting that some vaccines may contribute to autism, the number of parents refusing vaccines for their children, or demanding an 'alternative' immunization schedule, has steadily grown.

"And even though that paper has since been discredited, and scores of peer-reviewed studies have failed to find any link between vaccines and autism, the suspicion that vaccines are dangerous has stuck."[1]

Wakefield is usually described as a doctor or a researcher but rarely as a gastroenterologist, which is what he actually is. We're routinely told that in 2010 he was stripped of his license by the British General Medical Council and found guilty of unethical practices and fraud. What the media would like us to believe is that Wakefield is the maverick doctor whose work has been discredited throughout medical and scientific communities and only misguided, desperate parents support him. Every aspersion and insinuation has been made about his motives.

It seems that if it weren't for Wakefield and actress Jenny McCarthy, the model, actress, activist, and mother who recovered her son, Evan, from autism, no one would have ever thought of linking the vaccines a child receives to the development of autism. Incredibly, we're almost never told any details about Dr. Wakefield and his research.

There was one outstanding exception to this blanket silence on what Wakefield was really all about. In a six-minute interview segment talking with CBS reporter Sharyl Attkisson on Oct 7, 2009, Dr. Wakefield described how he became involved in this controversy:[2] "The first study was a case series, a report of the clinical findings and the histories of twelve children who had regressed into an autistic spectrum disorder. Eight of the parents of the children said that this was following an MMR (mumps, measles, rubella) vaccine. Our duty was not only to investigate those children to see if we could get to the root of their symptoms, in particular their bowel symptoms, their diarrhea, their pain, and their mal-digestion, but also to report their history." The doctors studying these patients reported what the parents told them about regression following the MMR vaccination. Wakefield said it was their duty as physicians. The study concluded that these children had a new form of bowel disease—one that had not been investigated previously. It said that it may be related to the developmental changes that occurred at the same time and it called for further study.

Attkisson asked about the charge that Wakefield had told parents not to vaccinate. He said this was wholly untrue. After extensive research resulting in a 250-page report, he began advising parents to give their children separate mumps, measles and rubella vaccines and to space them out. At that time, there were individual vaccines available in Britain. Six months after their paper was published, the government no longer allowed the use of single vaccines. The only choice parents had was to give their children the combined vaccine. Wakefield said, "So the attrition, the falloff in the uptake of the vaccine, can be laid at the door of the British government for withdrawing the option."

When asked if his fellow authors had recanted the finding of the study, Wakefield said that they hadn't. They stood by the medical findings of the bowel disease in these children. They did retract any finding of a link between the MMR vaccine and autism, which, Attkisson pointed out, was a misinterpretation in the first place since the study never said that.

Wakefield was clear that he and his fellow researchers had called for more research because of the possibility that there was a connection. "A possibility exists and it still exists and it needs to be investigated. So it was an unfortunate retraction. What was even more unfortunate was the way in which it has been used in a sort of public-relations exercise to seek to discredit the study, and it was false."

Next Attkisson brought up the charges Wakefield faced before the General Medical Council in Britain. Wakefield explained that this is what happens when anyone challenges the safety of vaccines. The government will "isolate and discredit them" as an example to other doctors not to do the same thing. He quoted testimony from the Vioxx trial in Australia. There were internal emails at Merck, the maker of Vioxx, that described how they would deal with any doctor who questioned the safety of the drug. Wakefield quoted the line, 'We may have to seek them out and destroy them where they live.'

Wakefield added that when Matt Lauer at NBC asked him if he believed there was a conspiracy against him, he quoted the Merck email and said, 'Matt, this is not an issue of conspiracy theory. This is corporate policy.'"

Finally Attkisson brought up the charges that Wakefield had his own conflicts of interest regarding the study he had done and that he had falsified the data. He called these charges "entirely false." When their paper was originally published in the *Lancet*, they had all followed the *Lancet*'s conflict rules "to the letter." He pointed out that the journalist who'd made those charges had attended the hearing and should have known the charges weren't true from the testimony. He said there were no charges of changing any medical records made during the hearing.

Attkisson ended the interview by saying that CBS would "post information that will let people make up their own minds where they can read about both sides of this" on their website.

This interview was legitimate journalism. Attkisson allowed Wakefield to explain what he had done and respond to the charges made against him. If every journalist covering this issue followed her example, the public would have been able to see that there were two sides to this debate. Sadly, the Attkisson interview was to be a lone exception in mainstream media coverage.

One month earlier, in September 2009, on NBC's *Dateline*, Matt Lauer had a report on the controversy over vaccines and autism that put parents like actress Jenny McCarthy up against nationally known vaccine defender Dr. Paul Offit.[3] Lauer, in an NBC video segment showing McCarthy marching at the "Green Our Vaccine" rally in 2008 in Washington, D.C., and in a voiceover, dismissed the possibility that any science supported the claim that vaccines were linked to autism. "With no mainstream scientific studies to support her views, McCarthy's influence is a real puzzle for scientists like Dr. Paul Offit, pediatrician at Children's Hospital in Philadelphia and a world-renowned expert on vaccines."

Offit began by saying that if people wanted answers about vaccines and autism, they should turn to the experts and not to celebrities. While the video showed him peering through a microscope wearing a white lab coat, Lauer was heard saying that Offit had been defending the safety of vaccines since the beginning of this controversy.

As proof that he had the science behind him, Offit said that there were now studies of "hundreds and hundreds of thousands of children who did or who did not get the MMR vaccine," and they showed there was no link.

Lauer pointed out that Dr. Offit has been vilified for his position on vaccines and autism, and Offit responded that even though "it's been pretty brutal," it really didn't affect him.

Lauer talked about the fact that Offit has made millions on a rotavirus vaccine that he helped develop. He asked him if this was a conflict of interest for him in defending vaccines.

Offit's response was a strong defense of his work. He said that he'd worked on his vaccine for twenty-five years and that it "has the capacity to save two thousand lives a day." This is what motivated him, not the financial gain. Now his work was to educate parents so they make the right choices about vaccinating their children,

On May 24, 2010, Matt Lauer covered Wakefield's work on the *Today Show* after the news broke that he had lost his medical license in Britain.[4] Lauer began by saying, "The doctor who touched off an international controversy by first raising a possible link between the MMR vaccine and autism learned this morning that he has lost his medical license."

Lauer then recapped how things evolved after Wakefield's paper was published in the *Lancet* in 1998, especially the presence of a man named Brian Deer. He said that Wakefield's small study had never been duplicated and this is what led Deer to investigate Wakefield.

Brian Deer was then shown saying that two years before the *Lancet* article, Wakefield had agreed to testify on behalf of parents who were going to sue the maker of the MMR over vaccine damage. According to Deer, this was never made public at the time of the publication.

The video then moved to a segment from an earlier interview Matt Lauer had with Dr. Wakefield. "In an exclusive interview last summer, Dr. Wakefield disagreed. He confirmed he was paid to conduct research on behalf of the plaintiffs but said it was for a later study, one that was never published."

Viewers were then shown the earlier interview where Lauer questioned Wakefield about these alleged conflicts. Lauer said that one of the charges Wakefield faced at the GMC involved the way he had obtained control blood samples to use in his research. Wakefield explained that he got the samples at a birthday party for one of his children. All the parents were medical professionals, and they'd given their permission for their kids to participate.

Lauer questioned the ethics of doing this. He asked if the children were paid. Wakefield called it "a reward for helping."

Lauer countered by saying that the GMC found what Wakefield had done was "unethical" and that his research had been conducted "dishonestly and irresponsibly." He mentioned Wakefield's new book, *Callous Disregard*, and said his supporters still stand behind him.

The next scene was of Wakefield sitting on the *Today Show* set ready to talk with Lauer. The issue now was the loss of Wakefield's license to practice medicine in Britain.

Lauer began by asking if he should still address him as "doctor." Wakefield said that they couldn't take away his medical degree.

Wakefield said he was not surprised by the actions of the GMC. He felt it had been "determined from the very beginning" and the ruling was the result of "the pressure that the government brought on the GMC."

Lauer, seeming to question why Andrew Wakefield continued to defend his position, asked him outright if he had any credibility left. Lauer listed everything that had happened to him since the publication of the *Lancet* article, including the loss of his job and his medical license.

Patiently, Wakefield explained that his findings had been replicated five times by researchers in different countries. He described this latest happening as "a little bump in the road," and he said outright that "the vaccine can cause autism."

And as Lauer tried to interrupt him, Wakefield announced that the US government had been paying off vaccine-injury claims that involved autism since 1991.

Without addressing this shocking revelation, Lauer focused on Wakefield's original study of twelve children. He challenged the findings, declaring that there were studies involving "hundreds of thousands of children" that disproved what Wakefield found. He questioned why Wakefield could possibly support the claim of a link.

Wakefield returned to the actions of the government. He repeated that the federal courts had been quietly settling these cases for the last two decades.

Lauer's only reaction to the very startling news was to change the subject. He said that doctors had told him that even talking about vaccine-safety issues had resulted in parents not vaccinating and children dying from vaccine-preventable illness.

Undaunted, Wakefield tried one last time to make Lauer aware of the cases being settled in Vaccine Court. It was to no avail. Lauer proceeded to end the interview without responding to what Wakefield had just said. Instead he asked Wakefield about his next move. He promised to continue his work, saying, "These parents aren't going away, their children aren't going away, and I'm most certainly not going away."

It must have seemed to be a good tactic to have doctors talk about the Wakefield controversy because a lot of news outlets did it. On January 6, 2011, Fox News published a report called *Stop Lying About the Autism-Vaccine "Link,"* and the author was their own medical contributor, Dr. Manny Alvarez.[5] He seemed to take the whole Wakefield scandal very personally, declaring, "The level of frustration I feel every time one of these autism stories comes out just can't be described."

Alvarez went on talking about his son Ryan's regression into autism, and he voiced his own questions about why his son developed autism. He listed the possible causes: genetics, a birth injury, medication his wife had taken while pregnant. Hannah Poling, the Georgia girl who had been compensated by the federal government in 2008 for vaccine-induced autism, was mentioned, but Alvarez said she had a "rare, underlying metabolic condition" that caused "features similar to autism spectrum disorder." He explained that her condition had been "aggravated by vaccines." He was firm that vaccines had nothing to do with the increases in autism.

At the same time he blamed Wakefield for causing parents not to vaccinate their children, he said that more unvaccinated kids hadn't led to a reduction in the autism rate.

Alvarez declared, "In my opinion, scientific fraud is one of the most lethal crimes that any person can commit. . . . for a doctor to knowingly publish fraudulent 'data' to support bogus claims for personal and professional gain is disgusting."

Viewers no doubt got the message that the medical community had rejected any possibility that Wakefield was right. Alvarez predicted that the true cause of autism would be found, and he added, "Hopefully, not by doctors like Wakefield, but by doctors who are really looking out for our children."

Dr. Alvarez seemed wholeheartedly disappointed that a doctor could have sunk to such a level of corruption and deceit as to falsely link vaccines and autism. Did he ever ask himself about what might be motivating the vaccine defenders? Did he ever look into their conflicts or the evidence in support of Wakefield?

Did Dr. Alvarez ever hear about Dr. Peter Fletcher, the former chief scientific officer in Britain who was covered in the *Daily Mail* on March 22, 2006?[6] The *Daily Mail* said that Dr. Fletcher had looked into the issue of vaccines and autism and found a "'steady accumulation of evidence' from scientists worldwide that the measles, mumps, and rubella jab is causing brain damage in certain children." Fletcher also revealed why the link wasn't recognized by officials. "There are very powerful people in positions of great authority in Britain and elsewhere who have staked their reputations and careers on the safety of MMR, and they are willing to do almost anything to protect themselves."

Alvarez wasn't able to find any science linking vaccines to autism, even though there are now more than one hundred and fifty peer-reviewed studies by well-credentialed scientists from leading universities out there that do just that. He also didn't believe that the case of Hannah Poling had anything to do with other children developing autism. Instead, Alvarez was content to label Wakefield a fraud and leave autism's cause a mystery.

It was amazing that those reporting on the doctor who's universally blamed for one of the biggest controversies in medicine never seem to focus on what his research actually found.

Parents came to him because their children had developed bowel disease and autism simultaneously. The parents said it happened after the MMR vaccine, but, incredibly, none of their stories mattered. Instead we heard about all the research that showed it couldn't possibly be true. And Wakefield's revelation that the US government had been acknowledging the link between vaccines and autism for years in court decisions was neatly ignored. It was clear that no one wanted to hear the details.

Charges against Wakefield continued, and, in 2011, the *British Medical Journal* formally attacked Wakefield's work, calling it "an elaborate fraud."[7] The American media was quick to seize on the news. There is no better example of the bias of the press than what happened at CNN.

On January 5, 2011, CNN's Anderson Cooper covered the Wakefield story. It was clear from the beginning that Cooper wasn't interested in Wakefield's side in this controversy because, as we were told, all the evidence was already in. Cooper began by saying, "Just hours ago, the *British Medical Journal*, the *BMJ*, did something extremely rare for a scientific journal. It accused a researcher, Andrew Wakefield, of outright fraud."[8]

Cooper went on to cite Wakefield as the person responsible for parents believing vaccines cause autism. He said that desperate parents were swayed by Wakefield's study of "just twelve children—that's right, just twelve children." Jenny McCarthy was also named as someone else responsible for spreading this dangerous belief. Cooper told viewers that Wakefield said he had found a link between autism and the mumps, measles, and rubella vaccine. CNN showed videos of McCarthy being interviewed and speaking at a rally in Washington, D.C. A 2008 clip of US Congressman Dan Burton, whose grandson has autism, was shown talking about the mercury-based vaccine preservative thimerosal, which he linked to autism—this after we were told by Cooper that "lawmakers also latched on to the research." Burton was shown saying, "We've had leading scientists from around the world come and testify before my committee who are certain that one of the major causes of autism is the mercury in the vaccination."

Immediately, Cooper informed viewers the autism rate continues to increase despite the fact that mercury was taken out of children's vaccines in 2001. He said that the scientific community rejected Wakefield's findings and that "ten of Wakefield's twelve coauthors removed their names from the paper." In addition, the *Lancet* retracted the paper because there were ethical problems and conflicts of interest involved and Wakefield had also lost his license to practice medicine.

Cooper solemnly announced that the latest blow against Wakefield had come from the *British Medical Journal,* which declared his work "an elaborate fraud that has done long-lasting damage to the public's health."

Cooper went on to describe those backing Wakefield as conspiracy theorists who feel he's "being vilified through a smear campaign." Cooper referenced the work of Brian Deer and described him as "an investigative journalist who spent seven years uncovering the bogus data behind Wakefield's claims."

In the face of all this, it was amazing that Andrew Wakefield would ever consent to an interview by CNN, but he did. Cooper, in a manner reminiscent of a tabloid reporter, said, "I confronted Dr. Wakefield earlier by Skype."

Addressing Dr. Wakefield as "Sir," Cooper referred to the charges made by Deer. He accused Wakefield of altering his patients' records and seeking financial gain.

When Wakefield tried to explain that Deer's charges were false, Cooper immediately cut him off, saying that these things were published in the *British Medical Journal*, as if this fact disproved anything Wakefield might be saying.

When Wakefield referred to Deer as "a hit man" whose purpose was to discredit him, Cooper began firing questions at Wakefield about Deer's motives. As Wakefield tried to respond, Cooper kept on talking, referring to Deer as "an independent journalist who's won many awards."

Wakefield had his own questions about Deer and who was paying him, but Cooper stated that Deer signed a paper "guaranteeing" that he had nothing to gain financially from any of this.

When Wakefield said that Deer was being backed by the Association of British Pharmaceutical Industries and that this group is funded by the drug industry, Cooper dismissed the charge, again quoting Brian Deer.

Cooper's treatment of Wakefield was like a police interrogation. He accused him of fraud. He said that his findings were disputed by the pharmaceutical industry, the AMA, public health officials, doctors, and journalists. There were people from around the world saying these things.

When Wakefield tried to bring up what was in his book, *Callous Disregard*, Cooper responded by saying, "Sir, I've read Brian Deer's report, which is incredibly extensive."

As Dr. Wakefield held up a copy of his book, *Callous Disregard*, Cooper announced, "I'm not here to let you pitch your book. I'm here to have you answer questions." Wakefield found it impossible to talk, and Cooper continued outlining how Deer had talked to the parents of children in Wakefield's original study. He said Deer discovered that Wakefield had falsified the medical records of his patients, according to their parents.

Wakefield denied that Deer had ever talked with the parents. He said that all his original findings were true. In response, Cooper began to cite charges made by Deer against Wakefield, including the fact that these children really didn't have regressive autism. An exasperated Wakefield tried to explain that he hadn't diagnosed them with autism. The diagnoses were already in their medical histories when they came to Wakefield. He said that experts at the Royal Free Hospital had reviewed their files.

Cooper, interrupting again, said that in some of the children, the signs of autism didn't appear until months after their MMR vaccination, not within days, as it was reported in the *Lancet* article.

Wakefield once again urged Cooper to read his book if he wanted to learn the truth. Cooper didn't give Wakefield a chance to continue. He said emphatically, "But sir, if you're lying, then your book is also a lie. If your study is a lie, your book is a lie."

Regardless of what Wakefield tried to assert, Cooper attacked him. When Wakefield pointed out that research in five countries had the same results as his first study, Cooper said it hadn't. Wakefield disagreed. Cooper then wanted to know how come health officials all over the world said his study was discredited.

An exasperated Wakefield could only respond to that by saying, "I suggest you do your investigation properly before making such allegations." Wakefield told Cooper the names of doctors who had replicated his research.

Cooper seemed oblivious to what Wakefield had just asked him and didn't respond. There were clearly holes in his charges against Wakefield. He hadn't done his homework, relying only on the *BMJ* article by Brian Deer. He hadn't talked to a single parent. He couldn't cite one thing Wakefield had written in *Callous Disregard* that he disputed.[9] It's hard to imagine how this could be seen as legitimate journalism.

Cooper raced on, making more charges against Wakefield. He accused him of recruiting his patients for planned litigation against the maker of the MMR vaccine. Wakefield asked to be allowed to answer. He denied having any ties to a lawsuit.

Wakefield did say that he was "an expert in MMR litigation" but that it didn't have anything to do with his research on the twelve children. Cooper continued to accuse Wakefield of doing his research for financial gain.

Wakefield tried to explain that there had been a research grant but that it had been given to the medical school, not to him personally.

The fact that ten of his coauthors had retracted the paper was proof, according to Cooper, that the research was "a fraud."

Wakefield's answer was simple. "I'm afraid that pressure has been put on them to do so. People get very, very frightened. You're dealing with some very powerful interests here." He then mentioned a whistleblower who'd given him evidence "that the British government had indemnified the vaccine manufacturer for the introduction of an MMR vaccine that they knew to be unsafe."

Incredibly, Cooper had no reaction to the stunning statement that had just been made about the hidden motives behind the government's attack on him. Instead, he went on, relentlessly trying to sully Wakefield's name, including saying that he was no longer a doctor. Wakefield corrected him on this point and alleged that the attack against him by the government is an act of desperation. He said they're becoming "very, very frightened."

Once again, Cooper failed to react to Wakefield's answer to his question. Each time he spoke, he tried to change the subject with yet another personal attack on Wakefield. At this point, he blamed Wakefield for the deaths of unvaccinated children.

Wakefield could only answer that he'd never said parents shouldn't vaccinate. Instead he'd only urged the use of separate vaccines for mumps, measles and rubella. He added that the British government ended that option.

It wasn't clear any longer why Cooper was even allowing Wakefield time to answer since he completely ignored all that he said in his own defense.

Cooper next had CNN's medical expert, Dr. Sanjay Gupta, join the discussion. He was equally uninterested in anything Wakefield said to defend himself. Instead, he merely picked up where Cooper left off. He again claimed that Deer had proof that the signs of autism had appeared before the children in the study received the MMR. Gupta could only cite what Brian Deer had said about two of Wakefield's patients in the *BMJ*. Gupta acted as though there was no disputing what Deer had written. He asked Wakefield how he could include patients who didn't show signs of autism at the time they received the MMR.

One more time, Wakefield objected to the charges made by Deer. He tried to get Gupta to understand that the study wasn't about the MMR. Regardless, these children had bowel disease, and no other doctors had taken those symptoms seriously. It had nothing to do with litigation or because their parents had made an association with the MMR. Wakefield said Deer had distorted the real facts of the study.

It didn't matter to Gupta that Wakefield said that parents disagreed with what Deer said about the onset of their children's symptoms. Gupta was not able to say that he'd talked to any of the parents. He could only cite Deer as his source, and hastily he affirmed that Deer said he really did talk to the parents. Gupta repeated Deer's claim that hospital records showed that in the case of several of these children, there was no bowel disease.

In response, Wakefield detailed how an expert pathologist had been brought in to examine the children's biopsies. The doctor had made the diagnoses not knowing anything about the patients. He also testified about this to the GMC, so Brian Deer should have understood the truth about the bowel disease in these children.

Wakefield tried to elaborate on the bowel problems he found. Nothing had been said about this during the questioning by Anderson Cooper. It sounded like a very critical part of the story. How did this relate to autism and the MMR? Gupta showed no interest in elaborating on this aspect. Like Cooper, he appeared to only want to talk about the charges made against Wakefield.

It was as if Gupta hadn't listened to any of the answers Wakefield had just given to Cooper. Instead, once again he listed the charges that Wakefield paid his patients and falsified data. Once again Wakefield said the facts were all laid out in his book. He asked him and viewers to read it. He even volunteered to send Gupta a copy so he could read for himself what had gone on. Wakefield said Brian Deer's claims were disputed by some of the best clinical experts in pediatric gastroenterology, who had examined these children.

Viewers didn't get to hear a response from Dr. Gupta. Suddenly, Anderson Cooper reappeared, hurriedly saying, "Andrew Wakefield, I appreciate you being on the program. Thank you very much."

Thanks to the combative interviewing style at CNN, Wakefield was never allowed to tell viewers what was in the paper. Cooper never addressed him as "doctor," only as "sir." He didn't introduce Wakefield as a gastroenterologist. Cooper showed no interest for the fact that Wakefield claimed specifically that the British Pharmaceutical Industries had funded Brian Deer.

Cooper appeared interested only in discrediting Wakefield and not allowing him to present any evidence to support his side. The only charges against Wakefield came from Brian Deer. Why hadn't Cooper personally talked to any of the parents who supposedly disputed Wakefield's claims about their children? Why did Cooper say he'd read what Deer wrote but never once stated that he'd also read Wakefield's claims as presented in his book, *Callous Disregard*?

Wakefield openly pleaded with Dr. Gupta to read his book. This is the most glaring evidence that all this was a setup. No one intended for Wakefield to make his case. It was clear that the plan here was to make Andrew Wakefield the fall guy in order to dismiss any link between vaccines and autism. The fact that Wakefield's work revealed a link between the MMR vaccine and autism meant that children were possibly being harmed by a product mandated by the governments in the US and the UK was never brought up. The reality that both American and British lawmakers had indemnified the vaccine makers meant that the pharmaceutical industry could not be held liable if a link were clearly shown and that it would be the governments that would be responsible was a topic that seemed far too dangerous to discuss.

Then on January 17, 2011, on ABC's *Good Morning America*, there was a similar setup. Newsman George Stephanopoulos reported on the controversy over vaccines and autism stating, "No reputable study has ever established a link."[10] Following this, he introduced ABC's medical expert, Dr. Richard Besser, who laid all the blame on Andrew Wakefield, saying that Wakefield's "small study" had resulted in fears about vaccines and a growing anti-vaccine movement.

GMA wasn't interested in what autism was doing to children. Instead, Dr. Paul Offit was shown saying that because of the claim that vaccines cause autism, children were getting sick and were dying. Besser added that the *BMJ* had labeled Wakefield's work as an "elaborate fraud."

Next, Brian Deer was shown with the words, "Brian Deer, *British Medical Journal*" at the bottom of the screen, which seemed to imply that Deer wrote for the *BMJ*. Deer accused Wakefield of criminal activity.

Besser said that Deer had disproved Wakefield's study and that he did this by examining the hospital records of his patients. According to Besser, Deer had evidence that Wakefield falsified their histories. Following this, Besser recounted the actions taken against Wakefield and cited the studies that disproved a link between the MMR and autism. Finally he accused Wakefield of fraud and said he'd damaged the efforts of the medical community.

After that damning start to the coverage, the camera switched to Wakefield and Stephanopoulos sitting on an NBC set.

Stephanopoulos began his interview with Wakefield saying that Besser had summed things up "pretty well." That didn't stop Stephanopoulos, however, from once again telling the audience that other scientists had rejected his research, his coauthors had recanted his findings, his research had never been replicated and he'd lost his medical license. Now the *BMJ* was saying, "Clear evidence of falsification of data should now close the door on this damaging vaccine scare."

After all this, Stephanopoulos asked him why anyone should believe anything he might have to say.

Wakefield patiently began to explain his side, denying Deer's allegations and making the claim, "We stand by the findings that we originally reported in the *Lancet.*" He continued, explaining the no one had retracted the findings of a bowel disease in these children. He started to say, "What we reported was the parental history of regression following—"

At this point, Stephanopoulos cut Wakefield off. He charged that Deer talked to the parents and that the records of the children didn't match what Wakefield said he found. Wakefield could only say it wasn't true; he'd never talked to them.

Unrelenting, Stephanopoulos said, "Yes, he did. I read his study. I read your book."

Stephanopoulos continued to hammer away on the topic, telling Wakefield, "The truth is the original records don't match what was in your study."

Stephanopoulos then recited a litany of all the things that proved Wakefield was wrong. The interview turned into an inquisition, with the same charges being repeated over and over. In turn, Wakefield could only repeat that his original findings of a new form of bowel disease in children with autism had been replicated. Then he added an astonishing statement that was completely ignored. "When I left the Royal Free [Hospital], we'd seen over a hundred and seventy-four patients with the same disorder."

Certainly that claim was worth pursing, but just like Matt Lauer had done at NBC, Stephanopoulos immediately changed the subject and began attacking Wakefield's motives. He accused him of telling parents not to get the MMR. He said Wakefield was being paid by lawyers and that he planned to profit from the patent on a separate vaccine.

Wakefield tried to respond: "That is wholly untrue."

Stephanopoulos: "That is not untrue."

Wakefield said again that it wasn't true. He denied he stood to profit from this. He only reported what the parents of the children had told him. This didn't stop Stephanopoulos from repeating the charges. Finally Wakefield told him all these things were false. He said he should check his facts.

At this point, one might wonder how many times Wakefield would have to say the same thing in defense of himself. He made it clear that he started treating these children long before any of them sought to sue the manufacturer of the MMR.

At one point, Wakefield told Stephanopoulos that his study had even been replicated at Harvard and at more than twenty other institutions in the US. Stephanopoulos said that wasn't true.

Wakefield even tried explaining how Deer had misrepresented the facts in what he wrote, after which Stephanopoulos again repeated how discredited his claims were.

"The weight of the evidence is all on the other side."

A weary Wakefield talked about the novel bowel disease he found and how his research had been repeated, with the same findings. He called for more research on the link between vaccines and autism. None of this mattered to Stephanopoulos. He said that the Institute of Medicine had investigated "every single study" and that they were convinced there was no link.

Finally when Stephanopoulos asked Wakefield if he vaccinated his own children, he said she that his older kids had received the MMR, but the younger two had not. He added that he was not against vaccines, but there was no proof that the current schedule was safe. Rather than ask him why he felt that way, Stephanopoulos talked about whooping cough deaths in California due to parents not vaccinating. Wakefield could only say that he had never made any comments about the whooping cough vaccine. His work had been with the MMR, and he cited someone he called "an international expert" who said the safety studies were "largely inadequate." This was why he called for single shots. He told parents to research the claims on both sides of this issue, because as he stated, "there are two sides to the argument."

It was clear from the beginning that Stephanopoulos had his own agenda, and it didn't involve equal time for Dr. Wakefield. This is something we're used to in the autism community, but it was especially obvious in the *GMA* interview.

When I asked Dr. Wakefield about what happened, he said, "Stephanopoulos had the American people believe that he had read *Callous Disregard* and that he had done so cover-to-cover. One only has to read yesterday's *MedScape* article to confirm this. His questions and his demeanor lead me to believe that, in fact, this was not the case. I suspect that as the truth behind this issue emerges, as it will, he and others may come to regret being part of the witch hunt. Their attention should be on the real problems of autism and lack of evidence for vaccine safety."

Stephanopoulos made sure we all understood how ABC felt; we were informed at the start that Dr. Wakefield's work has been discredited and that the *British Medical Journal* found his claims to be fraudulent, based on the word of Brian Deer. Dr. Offit was described only as the author of *Deadly Choices,* without any mention of the millions of dollars he's personally made with his rotavirus vaccine.

Dr. Wakefield tried time after time to get Stephanopoulos to understand that, as a gastroenterologist, his focus was on the bowel disease that he was finding in children who'd regressed after the MMR. These were healthy kids who became physically sick. They developed chronic diarrhea, constipation, food allergies, and encephalitis. They regressed into autism. Are we to believe that it's all one huge coincidence that normal children suddenly lose learned skills, become autistic, and develop bowel disease all at the same time?

It didn't matter. *Good Morning America* wasn't interested in what happened to them.

Several things emerged as the interview progressed. Again, it was never acknowledged that Dr. Wakefield is a gastroenterologist.

He was described merely as a "British researcher." Not once were we told how Brian Deer was able to gain access to patients' confidential medical records. This was ABC's very conscious effort to mislead people. We didn't get to hear from anyone who could support Wakefield, the inference being that there was no one to do this. So, why were none of the other coauthors of the *Lancet* story ever contacted? Stephanopoulos seemed intent only on accusing Wakefield of falsely linking vaccines and autism, and, therefore, nothing was said about the actual health histories of his patients.

To make this fair and balanced, why didn't *GMA* interview Dr. Jon Poling, father of Hannah Poling? Health and Human Services had conceded the claim that the nine vaccinations the young Georgia girl had received in a single doctor's visit had caused her regression into autism. That story received massive coverage back in 2008 by every major news source, including ABC.[11]

Why wasn't Dr. Bernadine Healy, former head of the National Institutes of Health, included? She had publicly stated on CBS News in 2008 that she didn't believe the studies had been done that would disprove a link.[12]

Why didn't Stephanopoulos have even one of the twelve *Lancet* parents from Wakefield's study on the show? This is really critical. The whole issue here swirled around the medical histories of these children and the charge that Dr. Wakefield falsified records.

Who was the "international expert" Wakefield cited who said that the safety studies are "largely inadequate"? Stephanopoulos never bothered to inquire.

During the course of the interview on *GMA*, Stephanopoulos said to Dr. Wakefield, "I read your book." In truth, as he repeated everything that Brian Deer wrote about in the *BMJ*, it became glaringly evident he couldn't have read *Callous Disregard* (or if he did, he totally disregarded everything Andrew Wakefield wrote about).

In *Callous Disregard*, Dr. Wakefield gave detailed descriptions of each of the twelve children who were the subject of the *Lancet* article. He made it clear that they became patients at the Royal Free Hospital when parents sought help for their children's bowel disease. It was not because they were referred to him by lawyers.[13]

Dr. Wakefield meticulously went over the charges made by the General Medical Council, explaining how they were not true, yet Stephanopoulos never brought up anything from the book.

If he'd truly read *Callous Disregard,* Stephanopoulos would also have known that Dr. Wakefield never claimed that his paper in the *Lancet* proved there is a link between vaccines and anything. It was about a novel bowel problem in autistic children, and he thought the medical community would be interested in the questions he was asking.

Dr. Wakefield devoted a whole chapter of his book to Brian Deer and his claims. He quoted the numerous charges that Deer had made about him and his work in print and explained how each one was false. He especially addressed the claim that he had fixed data on autism and that he had recruited and treated these children for litigation purposes.

Stephanopoulos never mentioned any of the disturbing things Dr. Wakefield included in his book:

> The British government knowingly licensed an unsafe vaccine.
>
> They failed to warn parents about possible life-threatening side effects.
>
> They intentionally had only passive surveillance for adverse events.
>
> They secretly indemnified the vaccine maker.
>
> They used false and misleading information to promote the vaccine.

Corruption, collusion, and cover-up, three things we usually assign to the actions of our Centers for Disease Control and Prevention, are also true for the British government. Dr. Wakefield wrote, "Children were the experimental marketplace." None of this was talked about on *GMA*, and Wakefield was never allowed the chance to bring any of it up.

We didn't hear about the inside source cited in the book (coincidentally named "George") either, yet he's a big part of the story. He's a doctor and a health official, and for Andrew Wakefield, he was the source for a lot of vital information on the measles vaccine trials.

News people never acknowledge that the medical community has everything at stake in this. They pretend that it's all just about the science and all the science says Dr. Wakefield is wrong.

Dr. Richard Halvorsen, another British physician, pointed this out in an interview with me, also in 2011.[14]

> We have to take a step back and wonder what is really going on here. To go to such extreme—and desperate—lengths to annihilate Dr. Wakefield (the person, note, not the science), some people must be very afraid, presumably, that parents might actually believe something that is blatantly obvious: that is that all vaccines can cause serious adverse reactions, including autism. By denying what is not only obvious but also supported by a wealth of scientific evidence, these obsessive vaccine protagonists risk losing the trust of all parents and destroying the whole vaccine program, the very thing that they are trying to prevent happening.

In *Callous Disregard*, Dr. Wakefield made the comment, "The evidence revealed collusion at the highest levels of the medical establishment."[15]

Self-protection is a powerful motivation, and this is made clear in the book. "[I]t was the UK government that was (and presumably still is) liable for SKB's MMR vaccine damage."

In *Callous Disregard*, speaking of his work at the Royal Free Hospital, Wakefield wrote,

> Ultimately, it took a group of gastroenterologists to recognize the significance of these symptoms, not through some preternatural wisdom, but through the diligent application of their training. A new syndrome was described and the findings replicated around the world. Erasure from the Medical Register is a small price to pay for the privilege of working with affected families.

In the case of Andrew Wakefield, the governments of Britain and the United States failed us when they refused to honestly conduct their own studies looking at bowel disease and autism for a common trigger. The medical community failed us when, instead of examining Wakefield's science, they attacked the scientist. And finally, the press has failed in their responsibility to report the truth. There has been a massive and conscious effort to mislead the public.

Wakefield had to be wrong. That was the only thing that really mattered.

For its part, the medical community tried to disprove any connection between GI issues and autism. In 2008, a Mayo Clinic study did just that. The journal *Pediatrics* had the story, "Incidence of Gastrointestinal Symptoms in Children With Autism: A Population-Based Study," which reported on a study from the Mayo Clinic: "No significant associations were found between autism case status and overall incidence of gastrointestinal symptoms or any other gastrointestinal symptom category. The study concluded that "feeding issues/food selectivity" were behind GI symptoms in autistic children.[16]

Important news sources in the US likewise reported on the Mayo study when it was released.

The *New York Times*: "Restrictive Diets May Not Be Appropriate for Children With Autism":

> Researchers at the Mayo Clinic reviewed the medical records of over 100 autistic children over an eighteen-year period and compared them to more than 200 children without the disorder. The scientists found no differences in the overall frequency of gastrointestinal problems reported by the two groups.[17]

*WebMD*: "GI Problems and Autism: No Link Found":

> Now, a new study from Mayo Clinic in Rochester, Minn., has found no apparent overall link between GI disorders and autism, although the researcher did find some individual GI problems are more common in children with autism.[18]

NBC *Today* Show: Dr. Nancy Snyderman was in Aspen, Colorado, but took time to appear on the show, saying "The findings are very conclusive: There is no link between illness in the gut and the signs and symptoms we see in autism."[19] According to Snyderman, limited diets led to problems like constipation.

The findings of this study came as a stunning surprise to many parents living with chronically ill autistic children. The study conclusions are also directly challenged by lots of previous research.

Five years later, in 2013, the connection was recognized. On Nov. 6, 2013, *WebMD* announced that research at UC-Davis found that yes, kids with autism did have more GI problems than typical kids do.[20]

The journal *UC Health*:

> Children with autism experience gastrointestinal (GI) upsets such as constipation, diarrhea, and sensitivity to

> foods six-to-eight times more often than do children who are developing typically, and those symptoms are related to behavioral problems, including social withdrawal, irritability, and repetitive behaviors, a new study by researchers at the UC Davis MIND Institute has found.[21]

Lead author Virginia Chaidez said parents of autistic children have continually said that their kids have more gut issues, but there weren't findings on how often this occurs.

This study was considered so important that it received an award as one of the top ten scientific advancements in autism for 2013 from the world's foremost autism advocacy group, Autism Speaks.

Parents came to Andrew Wakefield because of their children's GI problems. He studied them and found a novel bowel disease associated with their autism. He asked for more research. It took fifteen years for that to happen. And no one acknowledged that this was what Andrew Wakefield said in his original *Lancet* paper in 1998.

Whenever experts acknowledge that GI issues are associated with autism, they run the risk of endorsing Wakefield's work. That was abundantly clear in *Forbes* stories in April and May 2014.

On April 30, Emily Willingham had a *Forbes* piece called "Blame Wakefield for Missed Autism-Gut Connection," in which her contention was that yes, GI issues do exist for children with autism, and they're related to anxiety.[22] Experts haven't addressed this problem because of the work of Andrew Wakefield. It had cast a "noxious cloud" over anyone linking "autism and the gut." No one has wanted to look into this connection because of Wakefield's "MMR/autism/gut red herring."

Willingham chastised Wakefield for missing the anxiety-gut connection in autism, after all, as she wrote, he is "a self-described 'academic gastroenterologist.'"

As if to drive home the point, *Forbes* had a physician attack Wakefield two days later, on May 2. Dr. Peter Lipson, a specialist in internal medicine, wrote a piece entitled "Discredited Autism Researcher Chills Future Research."[23] In an attempt to validate what Willingham had written, Lipson accused Wakefield of falsifying data in order to link the MMR to autism. He referred to this as "junk science," and because of this, experts haven't researched this important area of medical science linking autism to anxiety and gut issues.

At the end of his piece, Lipson called Wakefield's work "abominable," and he added a personal note which demonstrated his contempt for Wakefield. He wrote this about what Wakefield said about autism and bowel disease: "Research that comes with a ton of ethical baggage, such as eugenics and experiments done by Nazis on prisoners raise important questions. In this case, it's not the ethical baggage but the outrageous actions by a single person, actions that have hurt real people."

For daring to say that the MMR vaccine caused bowel disease and autism, Wakefield was compared to the Nazis. That was a charge that evoked many images, and, for parents in the autism community, the idea of experimentation seemed more fittingly applied to a one-size-fits-all vaccination schedule for which no one could be held liable.

# CHAPTER THREE
# HANNAH POLING

*"And if it is ever shown scientifically that these kids were getting this terrible condition because of these shots, the federal government would be liable in court to provide for the health care and some cases, if they're really badly disabled, the support of these children for their lifetime. So this is a very huge issue, not just on a humanitarian level, but on a financial level."*

—US Rep. Dave Weldon, MD, in a CBS News interview, March 6, 2008

Hannah Poling, the beautiful red-haired daughter of Jon and Terry Poling, did something no other child up until that time had been able to do. When her story broke in 2008, she put a face on the autism-vaccine controversy. Her history included normal development until an immediate and dramatic regression following vaccination. What happened was typical of so many children in the autism community, but the difference in her case was that the government had recognized it, and, in March 2008, the story was in the news.

On March 6, 2008, CBS reporter Sharyl Attkisson covered the Poling case in the story "Vaccine Case: An Exception or a Precedent?"[1] Attkisson reported that after eight years, the federal government had "quietly conceded that vaccines aggravated a cell disorder nobody knew Hannah had, leaving her with permanent brain damage and autistic-like symptoms."

Attkisson interviewed a member of Congress, Rep. Dave Weldon from Florida, who is also a physician, regarding this stunning revelation. Weldon was described as someone who had "long been pushing the government to aggressively work to develop ways to screen for children who might be the most susceptible to ill effects from vaccines."

Weldon talked about his concerns regarding the Poling case. He asked what this meant for public health and cited the need to maintain confidence in the vaccine program.

And he added, "If it is ever shown scientifically that these kids were getting this terrible condition because of these shots, the federal government would be liable in court to provide for the health care and some cases, if they're really badly disabled, the support of these children for their lifetime. So this is a very huge issue, not just on a humanitarian level, but on a financial level."

When Attkisson asked Weldon about the fact that the government has long denied a link between vaccines and autism, he said that they really couldn't do that after the news about Hannah Poling. He said the government needed to come up with answers about autism, and they're not doing that. They needed independent research in order to restore public confidence in the vaccine program.

The story had actually broken a week and a half earlier. Journalist David Kirby had a story on the *Huffington Post* on Feb. 25, 2008 called "Government Concedes Vaccine-Autism Case in Federal Court—Now What?"[2] It was about a vaccine-injury case that attorneys from the Department of Justice and medical experts at the Department of Health and Human Services had quietly conceded. While Kirby did not name the injured child, it was the story of what happened to Hannah Poling. He had all the details.

Doctors agreed that the child was born healthy and developed typically until she went to the doctor at eighteen months.

There she got vaccinated for nine diseases at one time. Kirby said two of these vaccines contained mercury. Within days, she began to show signs of autism, including the loss of speech and eye contact. There were other problems like insomnia and non-stop screaming. Seven months later, Dr. Andrew Zimmerman, a neurologist at the Kennedy Krieger Children's Hospital, diagnosed her with encephalopathy and autism.

Kirby noted that the government said that the child had a pre-existing mitochondrial disorder that was "aggravated" by her vaccinations, resulting in "regressive encephalopathy with features of ASD."

What did this mean for the 5,000 cases pending in federal court where parents claimed vaccinations resulted in autism? Kirby expanded on the significance of the Poling decision. He said that while mitochondrial (Mt) disease is rare in the general population, a study published on the NIH site along with other research found that among children with autism, 10 to 20 percent of them had Mt disease.

Kirby cited a *Journal of Child Neurology* article, "Developmental Regression and Mitochondrial Dysfunction in a Child With Autism," co-authored by Dr. Zimmerman, and the claim that his research showed a large percentage of the autism patients studied at Kennedy Krieger had biomarkers for "impaired oxidative phosphorylation"[3] (Jon Poling, Hannah's father, was also listed as one of the authors of the article.)

Kirby wrote that children who have "(mitochondrial-related) dysfunctional cellular energy metabolism" could possibly be susceptible to regression if they're exposed to infections or immunizations between eighteen and thirty months.

There was even more concerning information in the *Huffington* story with regard to the thousands of claims of vaccine-induced autism. Kirby cited a survey of seven families with current cases in Vaccine Court showing each child had markers for mitochondrial

(Mt) dysfunction. Their histories were similar to the case the federal government had just conceded. Kirby speculated on what this could mean for the 5,000 cases pending in vaccine court. Would the government also concede a percentage of these cases? Could the government afford this? What would this do to public confidence in vaccines?

The use of the terms the government likes to haggle over, like "autism" and "features of ASD," seem irrelevant here. It boiled down to the fact that a normal child suffered damage from her vaccinations and developed the symptoms of autism as a result. Kirby wanted to know why she hadn't shown signs of Mt disease previous to receiving those vaccinations.

Kirby called for more research on this critical topic to answer the questions that the Poling case raised. He said we needed to know how vaccines were related Mt dysfunction and the development of autism. He called on HHS to study Mt disease to find out if it was the thimerosal, the aluminum or the three live viruses and to develop treatment for children showing signs of Mt disease. There was a chilling question in Kirby's piece: "And, if a significant minority of autism cases can be linked to Mt disease and vaccines, shouldn't these products one day carry an FDA Black Box warning label, and shouldn't children with Mt disorders be exempt from mandatory immunization?"

Kirby included a response from a spokesman at HHS which showed officials seemed oblivious to the Poling case: The official said that his department had studied the claim the vaccines were linked to autism and "found no credible evidence" to support it. Furthermore, he affirmed that the government had never concluded that vaccines cause autism in any case.

The article ended with the sobering words that the "big news" is that "the United States government is compensating at least one child for vaccine injuries that resulted in a diagnosis of autism" and that nothing could change that fact.

The events that followed the announcement of the concession of the Poling case were nothing short of bizarre. The government acted as if there was nothing significant here. They continued to deny any link despite what the DOJ and HHS had done. Media coverage added to the confusion.

March 7, 2008, ABC reported on Hannah Poling on *Good Morning America.* In the introduction, ABC said, “In an unprecedented settlement, the government says there may be a possible link” between vaccines and autism—in the case of Hannah Poling.[4]

Terry Poling, Hannah’s mother, was shown talking about her daughter’s regression into autism, and then news anchor Chris Cuomo said that doctors feel that vaccines possibly aggravated her pre-existing Mt disease and that her neurologist father thinks it resulted in her autism. Cuomo reported that her parents said it was a vaccine preservative called thimerosal that caused her autism. (He added that most vaccines hadn’t contained thimerosal since 1999.)

ABC acknowledged that this case was unprecedented and that even though Hannah did have this pre-existing condition, “there’s likely a connection between her vaccinations and her autism symptoms.”

*GMA* then showed Jon and Terry Poling and Hannah, along with their attorney. Jon Poling was asked what this decision meant to him as a parent and as a doctor. He said that regardless of semantics, it was clear that Hannah had been a normal child until she was vaccinated at nineteen months. She hadn’t shown any indication of a pre-existing condition. She became ill at the time she was vaccinated, leading to the development of autism and seizures.

The discussion then focused on the question of how many other children might be affected just like Hannah. Jon Poling said, “As other parents hear her story, I think her case is echoed among thousands of other similar cases.” He cautioned against anyone saying that this was just "a very unusual, odd-ball case." He said that after extensive research into every aspect of his daughter's illness, they found that mitochondrial disease could be found "in relatively high frequency in children who have autism." In his opinion, there needed to be more research into Mt disease. There is the potential to treat the problem.

Next Dr. Poling linked the thimerosal in the vaccines Hannah received to her autism. He found that thimerosal has been shown to directly damage the mitochondria of cells. As for all the studies officials used to disprove a link, Poling said that because they are large-population studies, they wouldn't be able to find "a small susceptible population."

Jon Poling then corrected the *GMA* anchor about his statement that thimerosal had been removed from vaccines in 1999. Poling said that because it was slowly phased out of vaccines, it was 2003 or 2004 before it was no longer in use.

Chris Cuomo next cited a statement from HHS saying that they've never concluded that autism was caused by vaccination. He introduced Dr. William Schaffner from Vanderbilt University and asked him to explain how Hannah Poling's case fit with the official denials. Dr. Schaffner called it "puzzling." He said, "It would appear that the court had made a decision in advance of the medical science. The science is not yet there, and we agree with Dr. Poling: We need much more research in this area."

In defense of the program, Schaffner announced that all his grandchildren were fully vaccinated. If parents were worried, they should talk to their doctor.

Schaffner incorrectly inferred here that Hannah Poling's case had been decided in a court, which was not true. ABC included Schaffner in this discussion no doubt because of his expertise as a doctor, but he obviously hadn't done his homework. "The court" hadn't made a decision. Medical experts from HHS, after reviewing all the evidence, concluded that Hannah Poling's autism was the result of the nine vaccines she received in a single doctor's visit. They evidently had been convinced that there was proof of an association. Finally, while Cuomo bought up "thimerosal," he never mentioned that it's made from mercury, a known neurotoxin.

What ABC didn't mention when presenting William Schaffner as a medical expert were his potential conflicts of interest. He's a member of data-safety-monitoring boards for Merck and Sanofi Pasteur and occasionally consults for Pfizer, GlaxoSmithKline, and Dynavax.

*TIME* reported on Hannah Poling on March 10, 2008, in the story "Case Study: Autism and Vaccines," by Claudia Wallis.[5] Wallis was skeptical about the government's decision and the science behind the claim of vaccine injury, but she posed a critical question that was never really answered in her article: "If Hannah Poling had an underlying condition that made her vulnerable to being harmed by vaccines, it stands to reason that other children might also have such vulnerabilities."

The *TIME* story also cited Dr. Judy Van de Water, an immunologist at the UC Davis MIND Institute.

Van de Water said, "Some vaccines, such as those aimed at viral infections, are designed to ramp up the immune system at warp speed. They are designed to mimic the infection. So you can imagine, getting nine at one time, how sick you could be."

She went on to say that there's some evidence that children whose immune systems are slow to develop are more likely to develop autism.

Van de Water worried that current vaccine schedules may be overly aggressive for some children. She suggested that parents who are concerned about vaccine safety ask their pediatricians to give fewer at a time. And she added that parents shouldn't vaccinate a child when he or she is ill.

March 29, 2008, CNN's Dr. Sanjay Gupta brought in the head of the Centers for Disease Control and Prevention, Dr. Julie

Gerberding, to ask her about the case of Hannah Poling. This discussion was entitled "Unraveling the Mystery of Autism."[6]

Gupta asked her if there was a difference between the terms "autism" and "autism-like symptoms." Gerberding said she didn't have "all the facts. "I still haven't been able to review the case files myself."

This was a surprising statement. The Department of Health and Human Services actually conceded this case in November 2007. The CDC is an agency under the control of HHS. Dr. Gerberding should have been informed immediately when this concession was made. Furthermore, the Polings held a news conference on March 6, 2008, that was covered by the major networks. It's inconceivable that Gerberding was unaware of the event. Three weeks later, when she was interviewed by Dr. Gupta, she still hadn't looked into the case. She did admit that vaccines can cause fevers, and, so, if someone had this predisposition, it could lead to an injury with "characteristics of autism." She cited "at least fifteen very good scientific studies" and the work of the Institute of Medicine—all showing no connection between vaccines and autism.

Gupta then asked her if she was "comfortable with everything that we know." That would seem to be a ridiculous question considering the only thing officials can agree on about autism is that their vaccine program doesn't cause it.

In response, Gerberding asked people to keep "an open mind about this." According to her, vaccines save lives; they don't cause autism. In addition, she cautioned that we're spending too much time looking at vaccines, and we need to be "looking for other causes."

Gerberding referred to autism as "a huge challenge" and said it was "much more common than I think anyone realized," which subtly implied that the numbers aren't really increasing—we're just finally recognizing it more.

Gupta concluded the interview by thanking her and saying, "We're staying on this." Smiling, Dr. Gerberding responded, "We're staying on it, too."

Gerberding actually moved on from this issue by 2009. On December 21, 2009, National Public Radio announced that Gerberding was leaving the CDC and had just been named president of the vaccine division at Merck.[7] *NJ.com* outlined what she'd be doing at Merck.[8] "She will be responsible for the commercialization of the current portfolio of vaccines, which includes Zostavax for protection against shingles and Gardasil for prevention against human papillomavirus. She will also plan for the introduction of vaccines from the company's pipeline and accelerating its efforts to broaden access to the developing world."

In a Reuters story on December 29, 2009, about her position at Merck, Gerberding was quoted saying, "I am very excited to be joining Merck, where I can help to expand access to vaccines around the world."[9]

Other than these outlets, no one talked about Gerberding's move from government to industry. In these stories, there was no mention of her adamant denials of any causal link between vaccines and autism. No suspicions were raised over the fact that the vaccine industry had benefited from her unwavering promotion of their products as safe and effective and her move to a top pharmaceutical company position.

April 4, 2008, CNN's Dr. Gupta interviewed Dr. Jon Poling. In a segment also entitled "Unraveling the Mystery," Dr. Gupta talked to Dr. Poling about Hannah's autism.[10]

Gupta said, "Her case of autism diagnosis was conceded by the federal government as having been contributed to by vaccines." This was a really remarkable statement, considering how many news sources described Hannah as having "autism-like symptoms." Poling responded by stressing the importance of this concession. Yes, her vaccines had resulted in her autism, encephalopathy, and seizures—the government said so.

This seemed to be hard for Gupta to deal with. He said that as a doctor, he'd been taught all about the benefits of vaccination. Now this link had been recognized. Poling agreed and said it took his daughter's regression to convince him it was possible.

When Gupta started to say experts believe that Hannah's case was rare, Poling challenged that view, saying it's "actually not rare." Gupta asked him if he still believed that vaccines had triggered his daughter's autism. In his response, Poling made it clear that while vaccines aren't the only cause of autism, they were for Hannah. Then he added a surprising statement about what he had found in his research: "[In] the other cases that were at Johns Hopkins, there were only a few like Hannah; then others regressed for other reasons."

Next the conversation turned to Gupta's two young daughters. He said he was planning on having them vaccinated, but he also asked Dr. Poling for advice on what he should do, based on his experience with Hannah.

Like so many people involved in this issue, Poling stressed that he was "pro-vaccine" but that he wanted to see vaccines that are safe. He called for "a grassroots movement among pediatricians in the AAP" to come up with safe, individualized schedules for their patients. He added that his oath as a doctor was to each patient. "We didn't take an oath for the public health or the greater good."

Gupta again promised to keep covering this issue.

Many watching the broadcast must have picked up on something that Dr. Gupta didn't seem interested in. That was the fact that Dr. Poling said there were other cases at Johns Hopkins that were like Hannah's. There were "only a few"—but isn't that something worth pursuing? Evidently not. It seemed best to foster the belief that Hannah Poling's vaccine-induced autism was a rare, once-in-a-generation accident.

The tone of Gupta's talk with Jon Poling was respectful and inviting. It was not like the abrupt manner he would use with Andrew Wakefield in an on-the-air interview three years later.

Vaccine developer Dr. Paul Offit also took notice of the Poling case. The *New York Times* published his reaction on March 31, 2008, misrepresenting the facts of the case.[11]

According to Dr, Offit, a federal court had ruled that vaccines had "contributed to" Hannah Poling's autism. Offit ran through the history of the Vaccine Injury Compensation Program. He said it was designed to compensate a victim of vaccine injury "quickly, generously, and fairly," something many people who've dealt with the program would dispute.

Offit said that everything was working well until "vaccine-court judges turned their back on science by dropping preponderance of evidence as a standard." He felt this is what happened in the case of Hannah Poling. He said it was her underlying condition that "contributed to her autism" and that an expert had convinced the court the vaccines had made her condition worse. "Without holding a hearing on the matter, the court conceded that the claim was biologically plausible."

According to Offit, the court had been overzealous in their judgment, and they intended to "err on the side of overcompensation." He didn't feel that it was plausible that the vaccines Hannah Poling received could have done this kind of damage. "The Institute of Medicine has found that multiple vaccines do not overwhelm or weaken the immune system. And although natural infections can worsen symptoms of chronic neurological illnesses in children, vaccines are not known to."

Actually Offit's piece distorted what had happened to Hannah Poling entirely, and, to their credit, the *New York Times* allowed the Polings to respond.

In a letter to the *New York Times* on April 5, 2008, Jon and Terry Poling corrected Offit's false claims.[12] Where Offit had said it took "several months" for her symptoms to appear, they said, "She immediately developed a fever and encephalopathy, deteriorating into what was diagnosed, based on the Diagnostic and Statistical Manual of Mental Disorders, or D.S.M. IV, as autism."

Where Offit had claimed that "a special vaccine claims court" had decided Hannah Poling's case, the Polings wrote that HHS doctors, not a court, conceded her case. They took issue with the fact that Offit called the decision "careless."

The Polings' letter described how difficult it had been pursuing their claim and the fact that it had taken six years to be resolved. They challenged Offit's view that multiple vaccinations at once couldn't overburden a child's immune system. They called his claim "theory and risky practice for a toddler's developing brain."

There was one very sobering statement made that should have gotten more notice. "No one knows if Hannah's mitochondrial dysfunction existed before receiving vaccines."

The implications here are chilling. Could it be that not only was Hannah Poling's autism the result of her vaccinations, but so was her mitochondrial dysfunction? This was certainly a question that no scientist could legitimately say had been asked and answered. No one had ever looked into the possibility.

On June 19, 2008, CBS journalist Sharyl Attkisson reported on the real significance of the Hannah Poling story in an astonishing article.[13] She said that it was not possible to make the claim that Hannah Poling was a rare exception. No one had any idea how many children with autism had the same "undetected mitochondrial disorder Hannah had." Attkisson furthermore said that the government had compensated vaccine-injury cases since the early 1990s "that resulted in autism and/or autistic symptoms."

CBS reported that "there were at least nine cases" just like Hannah Poling.

Why was CBS News the only media source with this story? This was about evidence that the US government had knowingly covered up. Why wasn't Sanjay Gupta talking to Julie Gerberding about these revelations?

Attkisson made it clear—the ball was in the government's court. A link had been shown. What were they going to do about it? She also acknowledged the fact that for years, researchers had been showing us proof of the link in scientific journals. What was Dr. Gerberding talking about when she told Dr. Gupta that all the science showed no link?

At the end of the story, there was an announcement of an upcoming conference that was to be held in Indianapolis with the express purpose of looking into mitochondrial disorders and autism.

On June 28, the *New York Times* put out yet another stunning report, by Gardiner Harris, called "Experts to Discuss One Puzzling Autism Case, as a Second Case Has Arisen."[14] At the same time experts were meeting to talk about the Hannah Poling case, evidence was mounting that she wasn't an isolated case. What Harris revealed showed the government was also concerned with damage control. "Federal health officials on Sunday will call together some of the world's leading experts on an obscure disease to discuss the controversial case of a nine-year-old girl from Athens, GA, who became autistic after receiving numerous vaccinations.

"But the government has so far kept quiet a second case that some say is more disturbing and more relevant to the meeting."

This was an amazing revelation. According to Harris, who had seen the case report, a six-year-old girl in Colorado had suffered a severe reaction after receiving a FluMist vaccine. Her health continued to deteriorate, leading to her death, after surgery and being placed on life support.

Harris pointed out that this girl and Hannah Poling shared the same mitochondrial disorder. While cautioning that vaccines may not be related to what happened to these two girls, he said, "But suggestions that mitochondrial disorders could be set off or worsened by vaccinations, and that the disorders might be linked to autism, prompted the meeting on Sunday and has brought the disorders sudden national attention."

Incredibly, this *New York Times* reporter brought up the same question that the Polings did in their letter: Could vaccines trigger the development of mitochondrial disorders in children?

The phrase "But the government has so far kept quiet" seemed to imply that the government may not be forthcoming on possible vaccine side effects. This is almost unheard of in a mainstream news report.

One of the scheduled speakers at the Indianapolis meeting was Dr. Thomas Insel, the head of the Interagency Autism Coordinating Committee, created by Congress to address autism. The *New York Times* asked for his opinion on the two cases linking vaccines to mitochondrial issues. He was quoted saying only that he hadn't heard of the second case.

The revelation that there was yet another child like Hannah Poling didn't seem to be of interest to officials from the Centers for Disease Control and Prevention. CDC official Dr. John Iskander said he knew about the second case but didn't intend to bring it up at the meeting. He did say that "this is another case that points to the need for better data on the risks and benefits of vaccinations in children with these rare disorders."

Monday, June 30, 2008, ABC News published the report, "Government Examines Link between Autism and Vaccines."[15] It was about the meeting of people from government health agencies that included the Food and Drug Administration, the Centers for Disease Control and Prevention, and the National Institutes of Health held in Indianapolis on Sunday, June 29. They met to discuss the link between mitochondrial problems and the development of autism. The article said, "At the heart of the issue for many specialists and concerned parents is whether vaccines—suspected by some people as being a cause of autism—might trigger mitochondrial disorders, which lead to autism." That was a riveting question. What if vaccines themselves caused mitochondrial disorder? This should have had the attention of all those working in the vaccine program.

Jon Poling was quoted in the story saying, "I guess I kind of feel like it's Christmas Eve. Tomorrow is Christmas morning, and, hopefully, those presents will be grants in the form of serious federal monies to look into autism and its relationship to mitochondrial disorders."

The tone of the rest of the ABC story was much different from the sentiments expressed by Dr. Poling. It seemed that a number of people went to the meeting intending to deny that mitochondrial disorder/autism was linked to vaccination.

Dr. Douglas Wallace, director of the Center for Molecular and Mitochondrial Medicine and Genetics at the University of California–Irvine, was quoted in the piece. "Parents have observed a time association between when their child got vaccinated and when they had a worsening of their clinical state, but just because two things occur at the same time, it doesn't mean that one caused the other."

The experts were lined up against the possibility that vaccines played a role here. Dr. Bruce Cohen, a neurologist at the Cleveland Clinic, sounded worried about the fallout from even talking about a link between vaccines and autism. "I think there is some potential of causing undue concern when one hears about situations such as the Hannah Poling case."

Cohen made it sound that even if there is a link, the greater good is served by vaccines. "But when we look at all the benefits of the vaccine program in preventing horrible diseases and horrible deaths, I think you have to take it all into consideration."

The ABC story reported that a study by the Cleveland Clinic had found 1,000 to 4,000 children were born with MT diseases every year in the US.

The piece ended with a troubling example of the six-year-old girl from Colorado. It said that federal officials were investigating this case where the girl "was hospitalized, had surgery, and later died."

"Her case offers more evidence, according to the specialists, that the potential link between vaccines and autism merits government research dollars."

Then on September 10, 2010, CBS News announced how much compensation Hannah Poling would receive in, "Family to Receive $1.5M+ in First-Ever Vaccine-Autism Court Award."[16] The story said it was "the first court award in a vaccine-autism claim." The $1.5 million payment was for "life care, lost earnings, and pain and suffering for the first year alone." Subsequent annual payments of $500,000 meant that over her lifetime, the award could reach over $20 million dollars.

Reporter Sharyl Attkisson made it clear that the Poling settlement had great significance. "It's unknown how many other children have similar undiagnosed mitochondrial disorder."

Fox News anchor Alisyn Camerota reported on the Poling settlement on Sept 12, 2010.[17] She called it "groundbreaking."

"Finally a court has said yes, there is a connection between this vaccine and autism."

She had Dr. Manny Alvarez, a senior medical expert at Fox News, as a guest. He is also the father of a son with autism. Alvarez talked about the fact that "this little girl did receive at a single sitting multiple, multiple types of vaccinations." He pointed out that she has an "underlying mitochondrial disease" and he noted that it's "a genetic disease that got exacerbated by the vaccines."

Camerota commented that officials had no idea how many other children might have the same condition as Hannah Poling. Citing the case of his own son, Alvarez said he was normal until around age two. He hinted that maybe "we have to test children a little more careful before we start giving them so many vaccines";

at the same time he reminded the audience that "no one is saying that vaccines really created autism."

This seemed to bother Camerota, who said it sounded like "very fishy legal language" for the government to say that vaccination didn't cause Hannah Poling's autism but that "it resulted in it."

While one would expect that Manny Alvarez would advocate for testing autistic kids to see how many have the same condition that Hannah Poling had, he didn't.

Camerota called this hair-splitting "fishy legal language." Alvarez was more concerned that "an avalanche of other people" might do what Hannah Poling's parents did and sue over vaccine damage.

Margaret Dunkle, great-aunt of Hannah Poling and herself a senior research scientist at the Department of Health Policy at George Washington University and director of the Early Identification and Intervention Collaborative for Los Angeles County, had published an article in the *Atlanta Journal Constitution* on August 12, 2008.[18] In it, she talked about the concession made by the government in her great-niece's case. She sounded hopeful that what happened to Hannah and what the government had admitted would lead to change.

She left readers with the solemn warning:

> A loud wake-up call from a beautiful little redheaded girl from Georgia has provided policy-makers with a historic opportunity to tackle critical issues of vaccine safety. If they fail to answer, what can I say?

Dunkle also had an interesting op-ed piece in the *Baltimore Sun* on July 11, 2011.[19] At the bottom of the piece, readers were told only that "she also has a family member who is vaccine-injured."

In her piece, "We Don't Know Enough About Childhood Vaccines," she asked a simple question concerning vaccines.

"How many immunizations does the federal government recommend for every child during the first two years of life?" She had a good reason for asking the question because she'd found some disturbing new research.

Dunkle cited a study she had found in the *Journal of Toxicology and Environmental Health* that said, "The higher the proportion of infants and toddlers receiving recommended vaccines, the higher the state's rate of children diagnosed with autism or speech-language problems just a few years later."

Hannah Poling's autism was the result of her being vaccinated against nine different diseases in a single doctor's visit, and this was a factor in what her aunt wrote. "The critical number is how many doses of vaccine a child receives. Why? If a vaccine is strong enough to confer immunity against a disease, it is important enough to count separately." For example, the MMR vaccine is a single injection, but it is meant to provide immunity against three different diseases.

This was not an idle question. As Dunkle pointed out, the federal government recommends a battery of thirty-six doses of vaccine. She listed the number of shots kids get when following the recommended schedule.

Dunkle went on to say that there really were no studies on the cumulative effect of so many vaccines given together at one time. "While testing is routine for individual vaccines as they are licensed, research on the both short- and long-term effects of multiple doses of vaccine administered to very young children during the critical birth-to-two developmental window is sparse to nonexistent." She also talked about mercury in the flu shot and the presence of formaldehyde in vaccines.

Dunkle sounded hopeful that this new study that had been published in a professional journal would have an impact. "This analysis is sure to rekindle the debate about vaccine safety."

But it didn't. No one was interested. As long as officials ignore new research and the media doesn't report on it, it's as if it never happened.

In fact, the *Baltimore Sun* story generated a strong response from Steven Salzberg at *Forbes* on July 7, 2011.[20] Salzberg, a professor of Medicine and Biostatistics in the Institute of Genetic Medicine at Johns Hopkins University's School of Medicine, chastised the *Sun* for publishing Dunkle's piece and another one by vaccine-injury researcher Dr. Mark Geier. He said that doing this "has given a platform to the anti-vaccine movement." He described Geier and Dunkle as "the voices of fear and unreason."

Instead of citing Dunkle as a research scientist, she was described only as an "anti-vaccine activist." Salzberg went on to defend the use of mercury in vaccines and to deny there was any science linking vaccines and autism. He criticized the *Sun's* attempt to be fair and balanced. All the science, he claimed, is in on vaccine safety. There is no debate. "When the subject is vaccines, presenting the anti-science, anti-vaccine argument has real, and harmful, consequences."

Salzberg suggested that if the *Baltimore Sun* wanted to make amends for what they'd done, they might print op-ed pieces explaining the benefits of vaccines. This would "re-educate parents" so they'll want to vaccinate their children.

September 19, 2010, Alisyn Camerota, at Fox, returned to the Hannah Poling case and asked about the strange finding that vaccines "didn't cause Hannah's autism but resulted in it."[21] She noted that there are 4,800 cases pending in federal Vaccine Court. She found a real-life autism parent, one Becky Estepp from San Diego. She introduced her as a mom who claims that her son got autism as a result of the vaccines he received. She said: "Estepp has spent ten years researching this, and she noted that there are a number of families who were also able to receive federal court settlements for vaccine damage as long as they didn't use the word 'autism' when making their claim."

Camerota quoted Estepp, who described the compensation program as "federal attorneys defending a federal program using federal funded science..."

Dr. Marc Siegel, a Fox medical consultant, was also interviewed, and Camerota showed her knowledge of the topic. "CBS News just did an investigation . . . that found that parents who used the words 'encephalopathy' or 'brain damage' won their cases. Those who had the same symptoms but used the word 'autism' did not win their cases."

Camerota said that HHS was "playing a semantics game here."

Right away, Siegel cited the studies that disprove any link between vaccines and autism, including one just out in the *New England Journal of Medicine* that had looked at a thousand kids.

As he continued his defense of the safety of vaccines, Siegel said something that showed he might not be that well-informed about the issue. He noted, "A lot of attention has been put on that. The question of thimerosal as a derivative, that's actually been removed from the MMR vaccine. . . . There has been no proof shown."

Siegel then told us how many kids' lives have been saved by the MMR vaccine.

Becky Estepp returned to inform Dr. Siegel that the MMR vaccine is a live virus vaccine and couldn't possibly contain something as deadly as mercury. She pointed out that her son had numerous vaccines that contained 25 mcg of mercury and that he received forty to fifty times EPA standards for mercury exposure.

Estepp raised concerns over the study cited by Siegel. She noted that the study seemed to show that thimerosal, which is half mercury, had a "neuro-protective effect on the children, which to me seems amazing—it's a neurotoxin. It's the second most toxic substance on earth."

After being corrected by Estepp, Siegel called for more studies and added that "even if an association is made, that's not proof."

The Hannah Poling case sent shock waves through medical circles. Many in the autism community hoped that the denials would finally end. After all, now there was an established connection. Two things that were never supposed to be related, vaccines and autism, were found to have a causal link. Things would have to change—finally.

Incredibly, it didn't really make a difference. Despite all the coverage by the big names in the news, the story died. Very soon after the 2008 announcement, Hannah Poling was no longer talked about. By 2010, the amount of the settlement got hardly any coverage except from CBS and Fox.

By 2013, whenever the topic came up in the press, it was as if the Poling case and its multi-million-dollar settlement had never happened. The press reverted back to citing the fact that officials deny any link between vaccines and autism. All their studies were proof.

How could so many officials and medical experts so willingly close their eyes to the truth? Was this topic so controversial, so dangerous, that it could never be covered in an honest and thorough manner?

Little was said in the media about genetic predisposition for vaccine injury after the Hannah Poling story faded away. Then, in 2014, several articles appeared in the *National Post*, a well-known Canadian newspaper. They were written by veteran journalist and author Lawrence Solomon. Two of the stories dealt with the effectiveness of the measles vaccines and the probability that certain children will be harmed by vaccines. On May 1, the story "Vaccines "Vaccines Can't Prevent Measles Outbreaks" was published.[22] In it, Solomon cited one of the most credible vaccine experts in the world, Dr. Gregory Poland, from the Mayo Clinic in Rochester, Minnesota. The stunning subtitle read, "Measles in Highly Immunized Societies Occurs Primarily Among Those Previously Immunized."

The story told about outbreaks of measles in fully vaccinated populations, and it went on to say that, according to Poland, immunity from the vaccine wears off after only a few years.

Incredibly, for someone with strong ties to the CDC and to Merck, Poland also talked about the possibility that certain children can be harmed by the measles vaccine. Solomon wrote, "The genetic predisposition of others makes them susceptible to harm from the measles vaccine, leading to public wariness, including among the well-educated."

*"Harm from the measles vaccine"?* Experts almost never acknowledge that possibility when they're promoting their one-size-fits-all schedule.

Poland had a solution to the problem of ineffective and dangerous vaccines: he was proposing the new age of vaccinology. The "next generation vaccine technology," which readers were told Poland is working on, would "personalize" vaccines to an individual's genetic makeup.

In another story on May 8, entitled "One-Size-Fits-All Vaccines Will Soon Be Replaced by Safer, More Effective Ones," Solomon continued his coverage.[23] The title itself was bound to raise concerns and lead to obvious questions: Aren't the ones we have now safe? Don't they prevent disease as long as everyone's vaccinated?

Solomon gave readers more insights from Dr. Poland at the Mayo Clinic on why we need to rethink vaccination. "Now measles is coming back, and it isn't likely to stop, not until old-school vaccine scientists give up their 'cherished dogma,' recognize the many limitations in today's vaccines and adopt twenty-first century thinking." A person's genes determine how they will respond to a vaccine. Poland believes that once the genetics of vaccination is understood, "science can identify what genes or gene combinations pose dangers in response to which vaccines."

All of this was shocking for those who routinely follow the pronouncements from health authorities in the US. Poland used the term "adversomics" to describe side effects. These are "genetically predetermined" according to Poland, and he wants to fix that. Knowing who would be susceptible to a vaccine reaction would calm the fears of "vaccine skeptics."

Poland's up-front recognition of the likelihood that some people will be harmed by vaccines is the Hannah Poling story. It's also been testified to by the eighty-three compensated cases of vaccine injury that included autism.

In the case of Hannah Poling, she was described as genetically susceptible to vaccine injury. Despite having no proof, health officials said she a one-in-a-million rarity. No one was interested in researching why vaccines led to her autism. Suddenly, six years after the Poling story first came out, a leading expert was talking about finding what might make certain people at risk for a vaccine reaction. While Dr. Poland said nothing about autism and vaccination, his research on "vaccinomics" and "adversomics" opened a door that could lead right back to Hannah Poling.

# CHAPTER FOUR
# SHARYL ATTKISSON

*"If vaccines can trigger autism in any way, directly or indirectly, that contradicts all the rhetoric and dogma heard from many public and government health officials for the past decade. And it supports what many other researchers have been saying for a decade, often to deaf ears, even after they published in peer-reviewed scientific journals."*

—CBS reporter Sharyl Attkisson, June 19, 2008,
on the vaccine-injury case of Hannah Poling

Over the last ten years, there has been one unwavering voice reporting on autism. Investigative reporter Sharyl Attkisson has done exemplary work reporting on autism as an epidemic and on the controversy linking it to vaccination.

In 2008, *Age of Autism* recognized her as "the best mainstream media reporter on the autism epidemic—breaking the news, asking the right questions, analyzing and synthesizing the data in a way that puts her slothfully incurious competitors to shame. In other words, she's doing her job, and doing it well."[1]

Not only has Attkisson reported on the controversial issues about autism on the CBS Evening News, but she's had even more stories posted on the CBS News blog. According to Attkisson, the federal government's concession of Hannah Poling's claim in the NVICP made a fundamental change in the controversy over the link between vaccines and autism. On June 19, 2008, Attkisson wrote an article with the title "Vaccine Watch" that made it clear that things were different.[2]

> [T]he debate has shifted from whether vaccines have any relationship to some cases of autism ... to what is the role of vaccines in some cases of autism. And how big is the pool of cases. If vaccines can trigger autism in any way, directly or indirectly, that contradicts all the rhetoric and dogma heard from many public and government health officials for the past decade. And it supports what many other researchers have been saying for a decade, often to deaf ears, even after they published in peer-reviewed scientific journals.

Attkisson stated what should have been obvious to everyone. If vaccines caused Hannah Poling's regression into autism, then there is a link. It's that simple, and all the rhetoric about "autism-like symptoms" and "vaccines resulting in her autism" but not causing it, as many news sources reported, is meaningless. Autism is diagnosed by its symptoms. There's no blood test or brain scan that confirms that a child has autism; it's based on the symptoms the child displays. If the child has the symptoms, the child has autism, and Hannah Poling does indeed have autism, according to her doctors and her parents. Most of the major news outlets were happy to let the Poling story die a natural death from neglect, and they hastily reverted back to telling us that the government has never recognized any vaccine injury that included autism.

In her 2008 piece, Attkisson pointed out something that entities like the American Academy of Pediatrics and the Centers for Disease Control and Prevention have covered up for years. There are researchers who dispute the official claim of no link between vaccines and autism, and they've been saying it for years; while their studies are published in peer-reviewed scientific journals, their work is completely ignored by the mainstream media and federal health officials.

Attkisson acknowledged the government's role in the cover-up and how much officials actually knew but weren't saying publicly. She wrote, "After a decade of denying any possible association between vaccines and autism, the government quietly settled a vaccine-autism case last fall. When news of the case leaked out to the public months later, government officials labeled the case of Hannah Poling an 'anomaly.' The truth is, nobody is in a position to know whether Hannah's case is an exception."

Attkisson said that officials told her the government hasn't investigated how many claims of vaccine-induced autism might involve kids who have the same medical condition as Hannah. Furthermore, they hadn't looked into the compensated cases of vaccine injury to see if these children had something in common that made them susceptible to side effects.

Then Attkisson revealed something that should have changed the entire debate over autism and vaccines, namely that there were "other cases that have been paid." She explained that over the last twenty years, the US government had been paying off vaccine-injury claims that included autism as a side effect. She said that after searching through government records, CBS News had discovered nine more where children with a claim of vaccine-induced autism had received compensation. All this was happening privately, while, publicly, officials continued the strong contention that no link had ever been recognized.

In addition, Attkisson noted that there were cases where the injury was "encephalopathy" that also involved autism, without actually using the term. Viewers were told that the government didn't track this information.

So it was clear, at least to Sharyl Attkisson in 2008, that the government was aware that vaccines could cause autism.

Attkisson continued to talk about the government's role in burying the truth about a link between vaccines and autism. In August 2008, CBS published her story "Learning From a Previous Vaccine-Autism Case?"—a piece that gave us more details about the Poling case.[3] She revealed that Hannah Poling's claim had been one of nine "test cases" that would determine the outcome for several thousand claims of vaccine injury that included autism. But the Poling case was never settled by a special master in Vaccine Court, because the government conceded the case outright. In the court records, experts had agreed that the evidence had shown that the vaccines she received "significantly aggravated an underlying mitochondrial disorder" which resulted in "a regressive encephalopathy with features of autism spectrum disorder."

This pronouncement came from the DVIC (the Division of Vaccine Injury Compensation, Department of Health and Human Services). HHS also oversees the CDC, the agency that adamantly denies any link between their vaccines and autism.

Attkisson went on to say that while this is the first known concession of a vaccine-injury case involving a child developing autism, there were other cases that went before the special masters and that the injured parties had won their cases. There were children with pre-existing conditions like Hannah Poling's mitochondrial disorder. Attkisson specifically cited a 1986 case of a child who had "tuberous sclerosis" or TS. "According to court testimony, many children with TS will suffer seizures and brain damage." The court acknowledged that the DPT vaccine likely triggered the seizures, and they agreed to pay for seizure medication but nothing involving the child's autism or mental retardation, because they were considered to be the result of the TS. Later, the court reversed this decision and covered all the injuries because it was determined that the vaccine had "aggravated the child's pre-existing condition" which led to the other problems.

It's clear that the NVICP understood that if a child has a certain condition like mitochondrial disorder or tuberous sclerosis, they're susceptible to vaccine injury. That injury can be encephalopathy and resulting seizures which can lead to regression into autism. The bottom line is that the vaccine is the trigger. This was undeniable, and it should have had the attention of health officials.

Attkisson ended her report saying, "One public health official recently told me that common ground on both sides might be a goal of finding out if there's a way to identify the conditions at play, screen children to identify those apt to suffer, and figure out how to continue a robust vaccination program that protects the nation but is also safe for potentially susceptible children."

While that sounded reasonable and responsible, it was never going to happen, because, if the government were to start screening kids for these pre-existing conditions, they would be acknowledging what the Poling case showed: if a child is vulnerable, vaccination can result in autism.

2008 was not the first time Attkisson reported on autism and vaccines. I saw her coverage back in 2004 in a CBS News report entitled "Vaccines Link to Autism?" She showed Jim Donnelly, father of Alex, who told us that his son was a healthy baby until he was vaccinated with vaccines containing the mercury-based preservative, thimerosal.[4] Attkisson pointed out that the flu vaccine still has mercury, a known neurotoxin, and that this was a concern to many people. "Nobody makes the claim that all ADD and autism cases are caused by the mercury in vaccines. But many researchers believe it plays a large role in our epidemic of the 1990s."

Next, Attkisson was shown with Dr. Mady Hornig, at Columbia University, whose research on the effects of thimerosal on mice revealed that they developed brain problems resulting "in all sorts of strange behaviors that were repetitive in nature, where animals would just keep repeating the same behavior in a very stereotyped fashion."

Attkisson further explained that these mice showed characteristics similar to those of autistic children, including repetitive behaviors, resistance to change, and social isolation.

The ending of this report was a direct reference to liability. Attkisson noted that while federal officials and other scientists don't believe that thimerosal can cause autism, "if it's true, hundreds of thousands of American kids could be living with the fallout. And the results could be devastating to vaccine makers and federal health officials who have steadfastly defended the use of mercury, a potent neurotoxin, in childhood vaccines."

Over the next few years, despite a great deal of criticism, Attkisson continued to report on the growing claim of a link between an ever-expanding vaccine schedule and the exponential increase in autism.

In 2007, she reported on Michelle Cedillo in "Vaccines on Trial."[5] The video coverage began with the scene of the twelve-year-old severely autistic girl lying in her bed. Attkisson stated what must have the unthinkable to many of the vaccine defenders. She said Michelle's case "could open the door for thousands of autistic children to be paid by a government fund. The controversy: whether their autism was caused by their childhood shots."

Michelle's parents were shown on camera holding a photo of their daughter as a bright, smiling baby, and viewers were told, "Michelle's parents say it was a month after this family photo that their world collapsed. Michelle got her measles, mumps, rubella shot... then ran a devastating high fever." Her parents explained the immediate changes they saw in Michelle. She was described today, ten years later, as "completely nonverbal," and the camera showed her confined to a wheelchair. Viewers were told that the Cedillo family's attorney would be arguing that the mercury Michelle got in her vaccines left her immune system unable to fight off the live measles virus in the MMR vaccine. Next, a representative from a pharmaceutical lobby group spoke, challenging the damage claim, citing all the studies that disproved a link. Attkisson ended the report by saying that Michelle's case was the first one in federal vaccine court to claim autism as a vaccine injury—something that more investigation would dispute.

Attkisson raised more questions on vaccine safety and the link to autism in 2008. She had an interview with one of the most prestigious names in medicine, the late, Dr. Bernadine Healy, former head of the National Institutes of Health and the American Red Cross.[6] Their conversation should have raised lots of red flags. A prominent member of the American medical community wasn't buying the official claim that studies showed no link. She was poised and serious. She publicly admitted that the science wasn't in on vaccines and autism. She said the correct studies haven't been done. "This is the time when we have the opportunity to understand whether or not there are susceptible children, perhaps genetically, perhaps they have a metabolic issue, mitochondrial disorder, immunological issue that makes them more susceptible to vaccines plural, or to one particular vaccine, or to a component of vaccine, like mercury. So we now, in these times, have to take another look at the hypothesis, not deny it. . . . Maybe there is a group of individuals or children that shouldn't have a particular vaccine or shouldn't have vaccines on the same schedule. I do not believe that if we identify the susceptibility group, if we identify the particular risk factor for vaccines, or if we found out that maybe they should be spread out a little longer, I do not believe the public will lose faith in vaccines."

What Dr. Healy asked for was reasonable. It made sense. It could be a way to restore rapidly eroding confidence in the vaccine program. What she didn't consider was how this would play out in the medical community. Hadn't health officials and doctors been adamant for years that there was no possibility that vaccines were in any way related to autism? Didn't they preach that they had the conclusive studies proving there was no link? Would they ever willingly change their position? There were a lot of children out there with an autism diagnosis. Even intimating that there was the possibility that for some kids it was the vaccines would be disastrous, and doctors knew it. After years of saying, "There is no link—vaccinate your kids," it was way too late to alter the message.

Attkisson persisted in covering this topic and focused on something that should have been a major concern for anyone reporting on vaccines and autism: What are the conflicts of interest of those who tell us studies show no link between vaccines and autism?

In July 2008, her story "How Independent Are the Vaccine Defenders?" revealed that this debate isn't just about the science and that there are plenty of reasons to dispute the objectivity of safety claims.[7] Attkisson reported that the vaccine manufacturers Sanofi Aventis, Merck and Wyeth had made hundreds of thousands of dollars in donations to the American Academy of Pediatrics. Furthermore, the industry also funds pro-vaccine nonprofits like Every Child By Two. Attkisson's report focused on Dr. Paul Offit, of the Children's Hospital of Philadelphia, a well-recognized vaccine defender who regularly gets coverage in the *New York Times* and on major TV networks. She revealed that neither the AAP nor Paul Offit would agree to be interviewed for this story, but she did have stunning figures about Offit's personal wealth. "Offit holds a $1.5 million research chair at Children's Hospital, funded by Merck. He holds the patent on an anti-diarrhea vaccine he developed with Merck, RotaTeq, which has prevented thousands of hospitalizations in the US.

"And future royalties for the vaccine were just sold for $182 million cash. Dr. Offit's share of vaccine profits? Unknown."

While there is nothing illegal about the pharma money changing hands, it is something that the public should be made aware of. Paul Offit is universally described as head of infectious disease at Philadelphia Children's Hospital, without any mention of his income from the development of a vaccine for rota virus.

Following the broadcast of this report, CBS received a letter of criticism from an industry-funded group, Voices for Vaccines, calling for a retraction of the report and asking them to issue apologies to the people and organizations that were talked about in her story.[8] It seemed that Attkisson had made her point and that the pressure was on to silence her.

In a written report on the CBS News blog, Attkisson released more information in a story entitled "The 'Independent' Voices of Vaccine Safety."[9] Congressional members like Senator Charles Grassley had found suspicious ties between the drug industry and nonprofits like the American Psychiatric Association.

Grassley was quoted saying, "I have come to understand that money from the pharmaceutical industry can shape the practices of nonprofit organizations that purport to be independent in their viewpoints and actions." The APA acknowledged that drug companies did have strong ties to medical organizations. The APA told their members, "We are not alone; recent public focus on relationships between medicine and the pharmaceutical industry is a challenge for the whole field of medicine." It seemed that the APA was siding with CBS, not Voices for Vaccines.

In 2009, Attkisson talked to Dr. Andrew Wakefield, the much vilified researcher who linked vaccines to bowel disease and autism in a paper published in a British medical journal, the *Lancet*, in 1998.[10]

In 2010, in a report called "Vaccines, Autism and Brain Damage: What's in a Name?" Attkisson reported on the semantics of vaccine injury.[11] She said that while vaccines were lifesaving, there was a price. "Certain individuals are injured by vaccination. The government understood this and had set up a federal compensation program to deal with cases of vaccine injury."

Attkisson went on to describe an investigation by CBS News that found there had been 1,300 vaccine-injury claims involving encephalopathy that were compensated by the US government. She said that in many of the cases, the child also had autism. Officials told her, "This was a separate issue," and they continued to deny there was any link.

Attkisson revealed that for many families this was the key to winning their case in Vaccine Court. Claims that linked vaccines to encephalopathy were more likely to win. Claims that said vaccines had caused autism were likely to be thrown out.

Attkisson specifically cited the case of Michelle Cedillo, which was one of the autism test cases heard in federal court. Although she had severe encephalopathy, her attorney argued that the MMR was the cause of her autism specifically. Her mother, Theresa Cedillo, acknowledged that using the word "autism," instead of "encephalopathy," meant Michelle could not win in federal court. She told Attkisson, "If you want to be compensated, I would stay away from the 'autism' word."

Over the years, autism has become closely tied to the issue of vaccine safety. It's almost impossible for news sources to report on the epidemic increase in the disorder without the comment section being filled with claims that vaccines are to blame. Despite the periodic official denials, the controversy just won't go away. Most stories cite the claim of a link to the mercury-based preservative thimerosal or to the live virus vaccine for mumps, measles, and rubella. Sharyl Attkisson has made it clear over the years that this is a very complicated issue and that it didn't involve just one vaccine or just one vaccine additive.

In 2011, in the story "Vaccines and Autism: A New Scientific Review," she explored the research of Dr. Helen Ratajczak, a retired senior scientist from a pharmaceutical firm.[12] After looking into the research on vaccines, Ratajczak said she believes there are a number of ways in which vaccines interact and cause autism.

Her findings were published in the *Journal of Immunotoxicology*. She linked the development of autism to damage from vaccines, specifically as it relates to the brain injury called encephalopathy. The dramatic increase in the number of vaccines our children receive can result in "the body's immune system being thrown out of balance," which makes children susceptible to side effects.

Ratajczak added a stunning new element to the question of vaccine safety: the effect of human DNA produced using cells from aborted fetuses or that contain DNA, proteins, or related cellular debris from cell cultures derived from aborted human fetuses in twenty-three of the recommended vaccines in the current schedule. This is a concern, as she told Attkisson, "Because it's human DNA and recipients are humans, there's homologous recombinaltion tiniker. That DNA is incorporated into the host DNA. Now it's changed, altered self and body kills it. Where is this most expressed? The neurons of the brain. Now you have body killing the brain cells and it's an ongoing inflammation. It doesn't stop, it continues through the life of that individual."

Attkisson asked Dr. Brian Strom, who'd been a government vaccine safety advisor on Institute of Medicine panels, for his opinion. He said he didn't know human DNA was in vaccines, but in his view, "it does not mean they cause autism."

Ratajczak didn't challenge Strom but simply asked for more research in this questionable area. She said that during her years working for a pharmaceutical company, she wasn't allowed to publish certain things, but now that she was retired, she was able to write what she wanted.

In 2011, Attkisson reported on a subject that wasn't in the mainstream news. In "The Search for Safer Vaccines," the public heard the sad story of a vaccine-injury victim named Elias Tembenis, whose case was successful in vaccine court in 2010.[13]

He was a healthy child until the age of four months. Within hours of receiving a DTaP vaccine, he began having seizures and then developed symptoms of autism. After his parents dropped the claim that vaccines had caused their son's autism, the government agreed that his seizure disorder was due to the vaccines he had received. Attkisson called it, "One more example where vaccine-injured children who end up with autism are quietly winning their cases, but only when they focus on the more general argument of seizures or brain damage rather than autism."

Sadly, Elias died at the age of seven because of his health issues. Attkisson pointed out the fact that his life and the injury he suffered should have some meaning.

She cited the need for "the right people" to look into this case to figure out why Elias suffered this injury. She reminded people that the former head of the NIH, Dr. Bernadine Healy, had asked for such a study.

No official seemed interested in investigating the 1,300 compensated cases. Attkisson ended the report saying, "What made these children get sick? Why couldn't they tolerate their vaccines when most kids can? Unanswered questions."

The chilling story of the death of fourteen-year-old Alex Spourdalakis, someone with severe autism, in August 2013, at the hands of his mother and his godmother, was covered by Attkisson.[14] She presented the background and named sources that provided a history of the case and insight into what drove the women to this horrific act. She sighted a documentary on Alex produced by the Autism Media Channel and quoted producer Polly Tommey saying, "Dorothy was like any other autism mother, desperate to get help for her child. His death didn't need to be. It was because there wasn't anything in place for him."

Attkisson described the out-of-control behavior, the trips to the emergency room, and Alex's mother's claim that severe gastrointestinal pain caused his problems. For almost two weeks, he languished in the emergency room at Loyola Gottlieb Memorial Hospital in Chicago in four-point restraints while his GI issues were left untreated. (The hospital was later cited for acting without doctor's orders in Alex's case.)

The report went on to say that after his stay in the ER, Alex did see a GI specialist who confirmed that his stomach "was studded with these lesions," too many even to count. Left with no insurance coverage or a facility to keep her son, his mother turned to ultimate acts of desperation—murder of her own son and attempted suicide.

Sharyl Attkisson has been a persistent voice asking the questions that no one else asks. She's attracted her share of critics for daring to bring up the topic. She has talked to the major players in the debate over vaccines and autism and has given us the details. Because of her, we learned about what experts like Bernadine Healy, Mady Hornig, Boyd Haley, and Helen Ratajczak have said about autism and vaccines. Her stories also showed us the parents dealing with the side effects of vaccination, especially regressive autism, parents like Jim Donnelly, the Cedillos, and the Polings.

She hasn't taken sides. She gives us experts on both sides. While most reporters downplay the impact autism is having, Attkisson has shown us the parents dealing with severely disabled children. She brings up the science that contradicts what officials are saying about vaccines and autism. Those of us in the autism community who follow this issue closely appreciate her tenacious reporting. We're left asking why more news people can't follow her example. And we need to consider the most important question of all about Sharyl Attkisson: Where would we be without her?

On Monday, March 10, 2014, it was announced that, following months of negotiating, Attkisson would be leaving CBS after more than twenty years. *Politico.com* reported that the Emmy award-winning reporter "had grown frustrated with what she saw as the network's liberal bias, an outsize influence by the network's corporate partners, and a lack of dedication to investigative reporting."[15]

*Politico.com* said, "She increasingly felt that her work was no longer supported and that it was a struggle to get her reporting on air." Her air time had been drastically reduced by CBS. Network news analyst Andrew Tyndall reported that Attkisson had only had fifty-four minutes of air time in 2013, after averaging two and a half hours each year from 2007 to 2009. According to Tyndall, she was "obviously being sidelined."

*Politico.com* went on to say that she is well known as an investigative reporter and was even called "Pit Bull" at CBS because "she gets on a story and won't let go."

Sources at Fox News were cited. Host Greta Van Susteren said, "She goes after the stories others won't go after, and she was right to go after them."

Conservative radio host Laura Ingraham was quoted saying, "She is actually doing what journalists are supposed to do."

Attkisson's determined reporting on the vaccine-autism link was noted in the *Politico.com* piece. "Liberal media watchdogs have tried to discredit some of Attkisson's work. Media Matters For America has accused her of 'shoddy, irresponsible reporting' and pointed to holes in her reporting on green energy and autism and vaccines."

In a March 10 *New York Magazine* story titled "The Right's Favorite Mainstream Benghazi Reporter Resigns From CBS," reporter Joe Coscarelli cited her "iffy anti-vaccine reporting" and included a link to a piece by Seth Mnookin from 2011 where Mnookin slammed her "anti-vaccine reporting."[16]

On April 3, 2014, Fox News reported on her move from CBS in a piece entitled "Sharyl Attkisson vs. CBS: Reporter First Tried to Quit a Year Ago."[17]

On the video with the story, Sean Hannity told the audience that Attkisson was leaving CBS News for several reasons, including what she called "an insufficient dedication to investigative journalism."

Fox contributors Tamara Holder, Ainsley Earhardt, and Kirsten Haglund discussed the treatment of Attkisson at CBS.

Earhardt noted that "it's odd that she hasn't been on. . . . It's very suspect when she's a top Emmy-winning reporter, an investigative reporter. She's known as the 'pit bull' over there at CBS because she holds on to a story, she runs with it, she doesn't give it up. It's true investigative journalism."

Holder noted that Attkisson is an investigative journalist who covers both sides of the story.

Hannity added, "Her stories weren't getting on the air, that's the point."

Haglund said, "It speaks to her credibility that she would rather leave and do something else."

In the print story, the public was told that the chairman of CBS News had tried to talk her out of leaving earlier and had promised that she'd get to cover more stories, but the airtime never materialized. Fox reported, "There is concern among some of the rank and file at CBS about the difficulty of getting management to approve tough stories."

Attkisson was on a number of shows describing how the stories she wanted to go after were all routinely turned down by CBS.

On April 10, 2014, Bill O'Reilly at Fox News talked about how CBS killed her reporting on the story about US ATF agents who allowed thousands of weapons to get into the hands of Mexican drug cartels.[18] The same thing happened when she began to investigate the Benghazi attack and Obamacare.

Attkisson told him some troubling things about network news coverage: "I think there are larger things at play in the industry. Broadly there are overarching concerns about just fear over original investigative reporting. There is unprecedented, I believe, influence on the media, not just the news, but the images you see everywhere by well-orchestrated and well-financed campaigns of special interests, political interests, and corporations, and I think all of that comes into play."

There are "larger things at play in the industry," and "unprecedented influence on the media," as we've seen when the issue is vaccines and autism.

On Easter Sunday, April 20, 2014, CNN covered the story. Reporter Brian Stelter on *Reliable Sources* questioned Attkisson about her reasons for leaving CBS.[19]

Stelter opened the segment saying that Attkisson had made "serious accusations of journalistic wrongdoing that involve one of the country's most respected news organizations, CBS News."

Attkisson talked about the forces influencing what is reported on in the news, including pressure from government and corporations. Executive producers, she noted, get to decide what gets aired and what doesn't.

Stelter made his own charges against Attkisson, citing "claims of a lack of accuracy and journalistic rigor."

In a one-and-a-half segment of this interview, Attkisson's coverage of the vaccine-autism controversy was discussed.

Stelter: "The loudest criticisms I've heard about your reporting have been about a series that you did years ago. It was about childhood vaccinations and whether those are linked to a rise in autism. You portrayed it at different times as a debate that was continuing to happen in the scientific community. . . . Do you regret those stories now, years later?"

Attkisson was adamant that she was standing by what she had written. "I think those were some of the most important stories I've done, and I would like to continue along those lines, at some point. It continues to be a very important debate."

Without bothering to ask why she still wouldn't back down on the issue, Stelter talked about the risks involved in discussing this topic: Parents might not vaccinate their children. She replied,

"There are many peer-reviewed published studies that do make an association, and the government itself has acknowledged a link." She told viewers to research this for themselves.

At the end of the interview, Attkisson gave this advice: "There are sophisticated efforts to manipulate the images and the information you see every day in ways that you won't recognize. I think we could all be more savvy about that."

It was very telling that Stelter said that "the loudest criticism" about Attkisson's reporting was over stories on vaccine safety and the link to autism. CNN has made a habit of one-sided coverage, including their attacks on Andrew Wakefield.

Stelter didn't seem concerned about the serious vaccine oversight problems Attkisson has reported on. Instead, he merely asked her if she regretted doing the stories. Attkisson's answer was short and to the point. No, she did not. There are peer-reviewed studies linking vaccinations to the development of autism, and the government has recognized the link in compensating vaccine-injured children who developed autism as a result. She would like to continue to report on this controversy.

And as she pointed out, this isn't just about the science. "There are sophisticated efforts to manipulate the images and the information you see every day in ways that you won't recognize."

# CHAPTER FIVE

# EVIDENCE OF HARM/ DEADLY IMMUNITY

*"If what I write in the book is all true, we have just experienced one of the largest medical catastrophes of our time and put a generation of American children at terrible risk with possibly devastating results."*

—David Kirby, *Imus in the Morning*, March 10, 2005

In 2005, after more than three years of work, David Kirby's book, *Evidence of Harm—Mercury in Vaccines and the Autism Epidemic: A Media Controversy*, was published by St. Martin's Press.[1] I had gotten in contact with David in the months before the book was release, and, like so many parents in the autism community, I was excited about the upcoming book. It was referred to by many of us as simply *EOH*, and it was well-researched and the information that Kirby had discovered made it clear that people in positions of power had some explaining to do.

Parents in the autism community felt that our issue would now be taken seriously by the medical community, federal health officials, and especially the media. All the trite phrases like "better diagnosing," "studies show no link," and "safe mercury" would no longer be regular features in stories about autism and vaccines.

In *Evidence of Harm,* Kirby asked some very concerning questions. Why didn't officials realize that the dramatic increase in mercury-containing vaccine paralleled the epidemic spike in autism? Why hadn't officials calculated the amount of mercury children were increasingly exposed to in the recommended schedule? Why was the mercury-containing vaccine preservative thimerosal, invented by Eli Lilly in 1930, allowed in vaccines when it had never been tested or approved by the FDA? Why had health officials met with vaccine-company representatives in a private meeting at a Methodist retreat center in Northern Georgia on June 7 and 8, 2000? Why was a last-minute secret addition, known as the Lilly Rider, included in the Homeland Security Act of 2002, barring any lawsuits over side effects from the high levels of mercury allowed in vaccines? Why did the Institute of Medicine report in 2004 that there was no link between vaccines and autism, relying solely on easily flawed and manipulated population studies while ignoring the mounting toxicological and immunological evidence?

Kirby's book provided the details on the deep pockets and vast agency ties of the vaccine makers along with the manipulation and cover-up of data by US health officials. There was so much evidence of harm in Kirby's carefully researched history of vaccine science and politics that I described it as the answer to the questions, "What did they know, when did they know and what did they do to cover it up?"

The media did give *Evidence of Harm* the notice it deserved. On April 17, 2005, the *New York Times* published a review by Polly Morrice.[2] Morrice acknowledged the stunning increase in the number of children with autism, the reports of children developing normally and suddenly regressing, the link between the MMR vaccine and gastrointestinal problems in children and the unanswered question from health authorities. "If this story has a smoking gun, it's the Vaccine Safety Datalink thimerosal study. Based on data collected from HMOs, this project, financed by the

Centers for Disease Control, sought to determine whether there was a correlation between the timing and amounts of thimerosal infants received in vaccines and the emergence of neurodevelopmental disorders, including speech delay, attention-deficit disorder, and autism. The Safe Minds statisticians contended that the government analyses of such data were flawed in a way that obscured or eliminated the original findings of statistically significant risks."

It was hard to ignore the all the findings on vaccine safety. On May 15, 2005, Gregory Mott at the *Washington Post* noted that self-protection was also part of the controversy.[3] "Behind the repeated pronouncements, from the CDC and elsewhere, that there is no known link between thimerosal and autism (which is widely understood to be a genetic disorder), the Mercury Moms see manipulation designed to protect against liability. The battle rages on, and while *Evidence of Harm* offers no prospect of a truce, it does provide crystal clarity."

*Evidence of Harm* was treated as a scholarly work. It was given respect. Kirby wasn't dismissed as anti-vaccine and dangerous, lacking any credibility. His work wasn't labeled a fraud.

Other reviews followed:

Knight Ridder Newspapers: "A riveting new book that examines this controversial but biologically plausible link, *Evidence of Harm* lines up the known evidence while telling the stories of a handful of determined parents forced to become their own detectives. You'll get eye-opening glimpses into the trenches where once normally developing kids slip into the shuttered world of autism and where their parents refuse to be bounced off the walls of seemingly impenetrable bureaucracies. Highly recommended."[4]

*Publishers Weekly*: "Engrossing . . . This is the book for concerned parents to read. It's accessible in its handling of medical topics and compelling in its recounting of the parents' fight." [5]

*Financial Times:* "Well-researched . . . This is an issue that will not go away."

*Newsday*: "*Evidence of Harm* is a gripping investigation. Much like the 9/11 commission's report, it is an alarming page-turner."[6]

*Journal of the American Library Association*: "*NY Science Times* journalist Kirby addresses the burgeoning number of US children diagnosed with autism, ADHD, and speech delays with as much detachment as possible, given what appears to be overwhelming, though anecdotal, evidence of a connection between those diagnoses and a mercury-based preservative. Some facts Kirby asserts seem hard to refute, and the juxtaposition of heart-rending parents' stories and disengaged rhetoric of official agency and company documents makes anything but refutation unconscionable."[7]

David Kirby was a guest on the talk show Imus in the Morning three times between March and June 2005, talking about his new book.

March 10, 2005: Kirby explained why he chose the title for the book, saying, "There's a growing body of evidence of harm . . . linking thimerosal to autism and other neurological disorders."[8]

Imus asked him why the CDC labels the kind of things he wrote about as "junk science."

Kirby acknowledged that people have "their own personal motivation for opposing this work, and it depends on who they are and where they work . . . The CDC recommended these vaccines very aggressively, and, starting in 1987, they started adding more and more shots onto the list without bothering to add up the total mercury burden that children were being exposed to." According to Kirby, the CDC "has some blame to share here."

Kirby continued, "If what I write in the book is all true, we have just experienced one of the largest medical catastrophes of our time and put a generation of American children at terrible risk with possibly devastating results."

What was most convincing to him, Kirby said, was the biological research done by experts like Dr. Boyd Haley at the University of Kentucky, Dr. Richard Deth at Northeastern

University, and Dr. Jill James at the University of Arkansas. These researchers had found that children with autism couldn't process heavy metals and that this led to their autism.

Don Imus questioned why officials would allow something as deadly as mercury to ever be in vaccines. Kirby agreed, noting that a vial of thimerosal comes with a skull and crossbones on it and side effects on the manufacturer's safety datasheet "are almost identical to the symptoms of autism."

Kirby further explained how the government had first become aware of the level of mercury kids were being exposed to and the increased risk for autism among those children. Because of documents obtained through the Freedom of Information Act, according to Kirby, the CDC knew that a clear signal of an association was there.

And these findings were not just something for Americans to be concerned about. Kirby said that we're also exporting mercury-containing vaccines around the world and that subsequently, autism is increasing, especially in poor countries. He added, "If you think they hate the United States now, just wait ten years from now if it turns out we've possibly caused this epidemic worldwide."

Imus and Kirby discussed pending federal legislation that would limit recourse if a child was injured by vaccination and would overturn state bans on thimerosal in vaccines.

At one point in the interview, Imus pleaded with his audience to get the book, calling it "wonderfully well-written."

Kirby explained that his book was written from the perspective of the parents of children who developed autism following vaccination. He went on to say that he tried to do a more balanced book; however,"a lot of people from the CDC wouldn't talk to me."

At the end of the segment, Imus talked about something US Representative Dave Weldon had said when he was on *Imus in the Morning*. According to Imus, Weldon had discussed what it would mean if the vaccine industry were held responsible for causing autism. He asked Kirby what the answer was.

Kirby agreed that someone was going to have to provide for all these disabled children, and he said the costs could amount to "trillions and trillions of dollars in caring for these people throughout their lives." Effective treatments were the way to reduce this burden.

April 4, 2005, Don Imus continued to report on, *Evidence of Harm* and again had David Kirby on the show.[9] Kirby began by appealing to both sides in the controversy over vaccines. Personal attacks served no purpose. He said, "I think it really cheapens the debate. We have a very serious problem and I think the kids are getting lost in it."

When Imus asked Kirby if there was a link between the mercury-containing vaccine preservative thimerosal and autism, he said that no one could definitely say there was or there wasn't. Kirby discussed the issue of ethyl mercury vs. methyl mercury and the claim that ethyl mercury was not as dangerous. He stated that both forms of mercury "attack the nervous system in a similar way."

Imus brought up the politics involved in this issue. He said that there were several bills in Congress that would indemnify the vaccine makers against lawsuits over thimerosal damage. He asked Kirby why the FDA had asked the vaccine industry to remove mercury from children's vaccines.

Imus also wanted to know what would happen if a link were recognized between thimerosal and autism. "We turn a bunch of crazy trial lawyers loose and bring the pharmaceutical industry to its knees?"

It was almost unheard of for anyone in the media to so openly talk about what autism is going to cost America and speculate on how we will provide for all the disabled children throughout their lives.

Kirby said, "We need to figure out a system. We need to figure out how we're going to compensate these families, how we're going to take care of these children, how we're going to remove the burden from the states—because right now they're footing the bill." He described how autism was impacting our schools and predicted that the costs were only going to increase. "My guess is the government is going to have to step in. And if, like you say, causation is shown, to prevent wildfire litigation everywhere, there must be an orderly way to decide who gets compensated."

During their conversation, Kirby pointed out that he hadn't been able to talk to any current employees at the Centers for Disease Control and Prevention because they weren't allowed to be interviewed. He explained that there is a database of reported vaccine injuries, but officials at the CDC "keep it under lock and key," in order, they say, to keep the information confidential. Kirby said, "I think the answer lies in that data. It's there."

Kirby said that researchers had looked at some of the data on vaccine injury and that what they say is there is very different from what the government claims it says. He called for an independent third party to investigate this information.

The discussion then turned to the numbers. Imus cited the current rate of one in every 166 children. He called autism "a national epidemic" and said "it's on everybody's radar screen." He asked Kirby what should happen. Kirby again said that we had to do something for these children and their families. We had to come up with treatments, especially ones to remove heavy metals.

At the end of the interview, Imus asked Kirby how he personally felt about a link between thimerosal and autism. Kirby said he'd be surprised if there weren't some connection.

Kirby pointed out the failure of health officials to address what autism is doing to our children. "If it's not thimerosal, what is it? Why aren't we in a mad rush to identify the cause of this disease and address it?"

June 17, 2005, David Kirby was again featured on *Imus in the Morning*, this time in a phone interview.[10] Imus started out by saying that the topic of mercury in vaccines and autism "is certainly worth talking about." The reason that Kirby was on the show again, Imus said, was because of the article "Deadly Immunity," by Robert Kennedy, Jr., that had just come out in *Rolling Stone Magazine* and *Salon.com.* Imus said that according to Kennedy, "If, as the evidence suggests, our public health authorities knowingly allowed the pharmaceutical industry to poison an entire generation of American children, their actions arguably constitute one of the biggest scandals in the annals of American medicine."

When asked how he personally felt about the article, Kirby said that Kennedy's stand was stronger than the one he took in *Evidence of Harm.* He said he was glad to see Kennedy's piece. Kennedy talked about the vast ties between the vaccine makers and our regulatory agencies. Kirby said he thought that officials sought "to disprove this theory," but he urged people to come to their own conclusions on the matter.

Kirby went on to talk about studies being published in leading journals showing autistic kids couldn't process toxins like typical kids. He said chelating these children to remove metals showed some had retained a lot of mercury.

Kirby said he hoped that the NIH could come up with money to fund studies to determine which kids are susceptible to environmental triggers.

Imus said he was going to have Robert Kennedy, Jr. on the show. Then he said, "[Kennedy] was scheduled to be on *Good Morning America*, and he was scheduled to be on *World News Today* on ABC. And he got cancelled. Do you know why he got cancelled?" Kirby wasn't sure about what exactly had happened to Kennedy, but he was told that it might possibly air.

As far as coverage for Evidence of Harm, Kirby said "I tried to get on every single program known to mankind." Imus couldn't understand why an author of a best seller who wrote about something affecting one in every 166 kids in America was being ignored by the media.

Imus compared this issue to "the whole tobacco thing, where no one wanted to talk about it for so long." He noted that US Senator Joe Lieberman had told him that the CDC "had a bunch of data" on thimerosal and autism that they wouldn't release. According to Imus, Lieberman couldn't get anyone at the CDC to return his call.

They then talked about how Chris Matthews at MSNBC refused to book David Kirby on his show. Kirby said, "His evasion was rather masterful. He did not want to talk about this." Despite that fact that he had a publicist who was "one of the best in the business," no one was interested in having Kirby on. He said that *The Today Show* interviewed him for an hour but used only a three-minute sound bite that made it appear that he believed there was no link between thimerosal and autism.

When asked about Kennedy's charges that the CDC was covering up data, Kirby said others felt the same way. He did note that there was the possibility of an upcoming Senate hearing where officials would have to answer questions. He said, "And if it's proven that thimerosal causes autism, we're going to have to work hard to fix it. We need to get to that step." Kirby again brought up the government's own data of reported vaccine injury.

In addition, in 2005, Fox 5 in New York did a story on the controversy over vaccines with mercury and autism, and they covered parents asking questions.[11] In this very balanced piece, Barbara Loe Fisher, from the National Vaccine Information Center, called for the removal of mercury from vaccines. Dr. Paul Offit countered, "Thimerosal doesn't cause autism." He cited the five studies that "have been done the right way" and which disprove a link.

The Fox 5 reporter noted that some experts disagreed, including Dr. Mady Hornig of Columbia University, who had found brain abnormalities in mice exposed to mercury.

Next, David Kirby was shown at his computer along with a close-up of his book, *Evidence of Harm*. Kirby said, "We don't have the answer to the main question which is, can thimerosal, can mercury in vaccines, lead to neurological disorders in a small subset of children?"

Viewers were told that parents had paid for a full-page ad in the *New York Times* publicizing Kirby's book. He referred to these parents as "smart," "organized," "motivated," and "angry." In addition, they have "lots of resources."

Advocates were shown meeting with lawmakers in Albany about a pending bill that called for limits on the amount of mercury allowed in vaccines.

The simultaneous release of *Evidence of Harm* and *"Deadly Immunity"* put the controversy out there, and Kirby and Kennedy continued to get coverage.

July 20, 2005, Robert Kennedy, Jr. was on the *Daily Show* with Jon Stewart. Stewart introduced him as an environmental attorney who's been speaking out on vaccines and autism.[12] Kennedy explained about the dramatic increase in mercury-containing vaccines between 1989 and 2003 and the subsequent increase in neurological problems in our kids. He listed "speech delay, language delay, dyslexia," and ASD, making it clear that we weren't just talking about one disability. He added that there was "overwhelming science" backing his claims.

Kennedy made it clear that vaccines for the most part no longer contained mercury, but he added that we're still selling mercury-containing vaccines to children in the Third World and that these countries are now seeing a dramatic increase in autism rates.

When Stewart asked why officials and vaccines makers continued to deny a link in the face of all the science, Kennedy said it was fear of litigation and of the possibility that a federal policy had "poisoned a whole generation of American children."

Kennedy talked about the reaction of the media to "Deadly Immunity." He said it was the cover story on *Salon.com* and *Rolling Stone*. ABC was all set to publicize it on *ABC Nightly*

*News* and *Good Morning America*, but just before it was to air, it was cancelled. Kennedy said he was told, "The order came from higher-ups at the network."

He added that after the network "was deluged with letters," they re-cut they interview, and what was broadcast was "virtually an advertisement for the pharmaceutical industry."

Stewart thanked Kennedy for his work, calling it "a remarkable story," and acknowledged the problems autism parents have to deal with.

Very important recognition for David Kirby came on August 7, 2005, when he was a guest on *Meet the Press*, hosted by Tim Russert.[13] What Kirby had uncovered about vaccines was getting attention. To answer for the government, Dr. Harvey Fineberg, the president of the Institute of Medicine, was also a guest.

Russert opened the talk with the essential questions raised by Kirby in *Evidence of Harm:*

"'Why did the Centers for Disease Control and Prevention (CDC) and the Food and Drug Administration (FDA) allow mercury exposures from childhood vaccines to more than double between 1988 and 1992 without bothering to calculate cumulative totals and their potential risks?' And 'Why . . . was there a corresponding spike in reported cases of autism-spectrum disorders? Why did autism grow from a relatively rare incidence of 1 in every 10,000 births in the 1980s to 1 in 500 in the late 1990s? Why did it continue to increase 1 in 250 in 2000 and then 1 in 166 today?'"

Russert asked him, "Have you answered those questions?" Kirby said that no one had come up with answers and that it was important that we do so. He explained how toxic mercury is and how much kids were exposed to in their vaccines.

Kirby's response definitely meant Dr. Fineberg had some explaining to do.

Fineberg showed no real concern over the increase in autism. "It's also clear that the definition was broadened markedly in the

1980s and 1990s, and there were increased incentives to recognize children from increased awareness and availability of services. No one knows with certainty what part of the increase is genuine, a genuine increase in numbers, and what part is from increased recognition of people who were already there but not previously recognized."

Fineberg's answer meant that if all the children with autism are simply because of "increased awareness," then the dramatic increase in mercury exposure in vaccines doesn't play a role. Fineberg next cited the population studies done in Great Britain, the US, Sweden, and Denmark, all showing no link between thimerosal-containing vaccines and the development of autism.

Kirby questioned the science. He said the epidemiological studies used by officials to disprove a link "range from severely flawed to seriously questionable." According to Kirby, no one was really looking at the toxicology. He said that when the Institute of Medicine studied the link between vaccines and autism, they placed "a preponderance of evidence or emphasis to the epidemiological evidence and rather, I would say, gave short shrift to the biological evidence."

Fineberg countered by saying that the IOM had looked at all the science carefully and thoroughly, and they were convinced vaccines didn't cause autism.

Next Kirby talked about the additional biological findings on ethyl-mercury's effect on the brain—things that weren't available when the IOM issued their report. He asked if the IOM would be open to reviewing the research. Fineberg didn't seem to be interested, saying "Most toxicologists believe that the ethyl form of the mercury is less toxic than the methyl form—less toxic to the nervous system. And that's based on many experiences with poisoning by these different forms of mercury."

Fineberg went on to criticize the use of chelation to treat autism. He called reports of improvements after removing heavy metals "anecdotal."

Russert brought up the meeting of health officials and pharmaceutical representatives in Simpsonwood, Georgia, to discuss mercury in vaccines and the increase in neurological disorders in children. While Kirby wouldn't say the government was involved in a conspiracy or cover-up, he did say there was "a lack of transparency." Fineberg strongly disagreed and said that he believed all the necessary information is available.

Kirby called for more studies and especially for officials to listen to parents whose children were born healthy and then regressed, while Fineberg had no doubts—"the best evidence all points to the lack of an association."

In 2006, David Kirby was on the Barry Nolan Show, and, in the introduction, the audience was told that they were going to discuss the claim of a connection between thimerosal and higher rates of neurological problems in children, and "the behind-closed-doors moves made by the US government to shield the holder of the thimerosal patent from lawsuits."[14]

Kirby began by calling for transparency in the vaccine program, which he called "a very important part of our public health policy." He said that parents need to have trust in the vaccine program. "The more the government levels with us, the better parents will feel about vaccinating their children."

They talked about the increase in the numbers, and Kirby said that he believed the increase was real and that it's impossible to have "a genetic epidemic."

Kirby went on to talk about the amount of mercury children in the 1990s received in their vaccines, which was way above EPA levels.

He also noted that the epidemiological studies used to show no link between vaccines and autism are not valid proof. The famous

Denmark study, according to Kirby, was deeply flawed because they changed the criteria in the middle of the study to make any association disappear.

Kirby was asked about the use of mercury in vaccines given to children in the Third World, and he responded by saying that these countries can't afford the more expensive vaccines that have the mercury removed. He brought up the obvious contradiction in our move to protect American children by removing thimerosal from vaccines while continuing to export mercury-containing vaccines to other countries.

The second half of Barry Nolan's show had vaccine developer Dr. Paul Offit's side in the debate. His support for the safety of thimerosal in vaccines was absolute. Offit began by citing the population studies comparing children who received either different levels of thimerosal or no vaccines at all. He said the results showed no causation between thimerosal and autism. He added, "Frankly, it never made biological sense that it would. There's really a wealth of biological data that I think looks at this question."

According to Offit, if a toxic insult was going to cause autism, it happens before birth.

Furthermore, Offit said that pregnant women who were exposed to methyl-mercury might have babies with seizures and mental retardation but not autism.

Offit wasn't too concerned about the current autism rate of one in 166. He was confident that it was due to a broader definition of the term "autism."

If there was a link between vaccines and autism at a rate of one in 166, Offit said that retrospective studies would have picked up this clear marker. The fact that they haven't is proof of no link.

When he was asked if genetics could predispose certain children to become autistic after vaccination with mercury, Offit was cited that "good epidemiological studies" disproved this.

If the environment does play a role, Offit said we should look for possible triggers—other things besides vaccines.

Offit said he was against the removal of mercury from vaccines. He said that even if they removed all the thimerosal from vaccines, if wouldn't affect the autism rate. In addition , according to Offit, it would be expensive, and doing so could threaten the vaccine supply.

A caller to the Barry Nolan show asked Offit if the vaccine makers were suppressing studies, and Offit told her that vaccines are made in order to make kids "safer and healthier."

Nothing was said in the introduction about the fact that Paul Offit wasn't just an infectious disease expert from Philadelphia Children's Hospital. The audience wasn't told about his financial gain from the development of a rotavirus vaccine. During his remarks, Offit referenced a comparison study of children who received thimerosal-containing vaccines and children who received no vaccines. No one has ever published this research. Parents have asked for comparison studies of vaccinated and unvaccinated children for years. It's hard to believe that Offit was privy to science that has never been shown to anyone else.

On Oct. 19, 2007, Robert Kennedy, Jr. was on the Joe Scarborough Show.[15] Kennedy said that today's children were injected with 400 times the level of mercury that the FDA/EPA considers safe. Scarborough acknowledged that his son had Asperger's Syndrome, a high-functioning type of autism.

Kennedy's message was to the point: "The science is out there today for anyone who bothers to read it." He cited the "hundreds and hundreds of studies" linking mercury-containing vaccines to neuro-developmental disorders.

When Kennedy was asked why the people involved weren't speaking out, he said it was because they're "now trying to cover their tracks." He talked about the "secret meeting" in Simpsonwood, Georgia, in 2000 where US health officials and scientists discussed what thimerosal was doing to children. He called the transcript of the meeting, "one of the most horrifying things that you can read."

On March 6, 2008, in their coverage of the government's concession in the Hannah Poling case, CNN cited David Kirby.[16]

The news anchor began the segment discounting any connection between vaccines and autism. "Government health experts insist there is no link between vaccines and autism, but they've made a major concession—not a ruling—in the case of a nine-year-old girl from Georgia. They conceded that childhood vaccines ultimately led Hannah Poling to develop autism." The anchor went on to describe her "pre-existing condition" that was "aggravated" by her vaccines.

There was coverage of Hannah Poling's parents during a press conference talking about the impact of all the vaccines their daughter received in a single doctor's visit. Her mother said, "I wanted to know why my daughter, who had been completely normal until getting nine vaccines in one day, was suddenly no longer there, no longer verbal, no longer responding."

Next, Kirby was shown in the CNN studio, described as someone "who has reported extensively on autism for *Huffington* and the *New York Times*." Also included in the coverage was Dr. Chip Harbaugh, member of the National American Academy of Pediatrics. Harbaugh spoke first and affirmed that "vaccines are still safe." He cited the studies that disprove any link. He called the Poling story "confusing" and talked about her "genetic disorder" and "pre-existing condition." His patients with Mt disease "look like they could be autistic, but they're not so."

When it was David Kirby's turn to talk, he called the Poling concession "very significant." He said that mitochondrial problems could affect as many as twenty percent of autistic children. The real problem, he felt, was that HHS wasn't willing to talk about it. He advised parents to look for information and "work out a schedule you're comfortable with."

Kirby made a statement that Dr. Harbaugh needed to take note of. He said, "Seventy-five percent of mitochondrial disorders are actually acquired through drugs and other toxins." If that was really true, in light of the Poling case, it could have serious implications.

Harbaugh countered by saying that mercury was removed from vaccines in 2001, and autism rates continue to increase. He explained that all the autism was because "pediatricians are better nationally at diagnosing autism." Plus, he said that the spectrum has been expanded.

The issue remained a heated one, although mainstream medicine and government officials acted as if nothing new had happened. Still, the subject continued to get coverage by the media.

On April 2, 2008, David Kirby and activist mom Jenny McCarthy were *on Larry King Live.*[17] McCarthy started by describing her son Evan's history of autism and seizures following vaccination when he was two. She talked about the autism community of parents and doctors that she had discovered on the Internet. She made it clear that she was not anti-vaccine even though she questioned the current vaccination schedule.

She made stunning statements like, "The way I treated Evan, the way a lot of parents are treating their kids, is not treating autism. We are treating vaccine injury, and the kids are getting better."

McCarthy asked for the science behind a tripling of the vaccine schedule since 1983. She alleged that there was a real connection between the increase in the number of vaccines children get and the epidemic rate of autism. She noted that there are "parent after parent after parent" who claim their child was fine until they were vaccinated. "They got a fever, they stopped speaking, and then they became autistic."

David Kirby was introduced as the author of "a provocative *New York Times* best seller, *Evidence of Harm*, who first became interested in this issue when a rider was added to the Homeland

Security Act of 2002 that would dismiss lawsuits against vaccine makers for damage from the mercury in vaccines."

Kirby made a dramatic statement about the link between vaccines and autism. He said, "We're here to discuss this debate whether vaccines are related to autism or not. I'm here, I've never said this before, Larry, this debate is over. Vaccines can trigger autism. It happened to Hannah Poling. It happened to many other kids. I confirmed it, and we need to deal with it." He added that there were lots of kids just like Hannah Poling out there.

McCarthy admitted that there were other things that triggered autism besides immunizations, but she felt that "vaccines play the largest role right now." She called for testing children for health problems and changing the mandated schedule.

Kirby talked about the impact of Hannah Poling and raised questions about mitochondrial dysfunction. He said we need to find out how many other kids are like this. Plus, he wanted to know what was causing these mitochondrial problems. Toxins were possible triggers.

When Larry King asked them about being anti-vaccine, McCarthy strongly disagreed but called for a vaccine schedule that is *"individualized to the child."*

Kirby described himself as "pro-vaccine," and he said was often criticized for having this position.

The big criticism of a show covering this topic was that it made parents afraid to vaccinate. McCarthy told Larry King that parents not vaccinating is "the only thing that's going to shake up the CDC to do something about it."

The Centers for Disease Control and Prevention had sent a statement to Larry King, which he read. It said that parents shouldn't be worried about vaccinating their children because "the current recommendations to vaccinate are based on years of scientific research by the world's foremost experts." Parents were also told to talk to their child's doctor.

McCarthy brought up the fact that for many parents, "our trust is broken" because doctors haven't been listening to parents.

In the next segment, Kirby and McCarthy were joined by McCarthy's son's doctor, Jay Gordon, MD, associate professor of pediatrics at UCLA Medical School, who had recently put out a DVD called *Vaccinations: Assessing the Risks and the Benefits,* Harvey Karp, MD, author of *The Happiest Toddler on the Block* and member of the American Academy of Pediatrics, and president elect of the AAP, David Tayloe, MD. As part of his introductions, King said neither Karp nor Tayloe believed vaccines can cause autism.

Dr. Karp talked about all the studies disproving any link between vaccines and autism. He even went so far as to say, "Kids that have autism don't usually have an immunization that occurs right before the onset of their symptoms."

Dr. Tayloe began his comments attesting to the benefits of vaccination and the need for herd immunity. He said in his practice he'd never had a child he referred to the compensation program for vaccine injury.

When Kirby asked if the AAP would support a current bill in Congress that called for a study of vaccinated vs. unvaccinated children, Tayloe responded by saying, "We're not afraid of the truth at the American Academy of Pediatrics," but he did not specifically answer the question.

In some ways, it was a sparring match between the doctors, with Tayloe and Karp on one side and Gordon on the other. At one point, Dr. Gordon pointed out that David Kirby's book was called *Evidence of Harm,* and he was adamant that "the evidence is there." According to Gordon, there were flaws in the one-size-fits-all vaccination schedule, and officials weren't doing anything about it.

In the April/May 2008 issue of *SPECTRUM,* a magazine for families and individuals with autism and developmental disabilities, Robert Kennedy, Jr. described what it's like dealing with the *New York Times* when the subject is autism.[18] In the article "RFK Jr., His Crusade Continues," by Sarah Bridges, PhD, readers were told about a meeting that was supposed to include Kennedy and the editor at the *Times* to discuss Kennedy's editorial submission on vaccines and autism in 2006.

Kennedy was accompanied by Dr. Boyd Haley, chairman of the chemistry department at the University of Kentucky and an expert in mercury toxicity. What should have been an open exchange with a *Times* editor turned into a confrontation. Kennedy and Haley found themselves facing a whole room filled with hostile staff members.

Kennedy said that it was like "talking to a brick wall. They were absolutely determined that there would be no public discussion in their paper about mercury and neurological disorders."

According to Bridges, no one at the *Times* cared how much evidence Haley and Kennedy had with them. They stuck by the mantra, "The CDC says the vaccines are safe."

Kennedy summed it up well: "The unbelievable thing is how these children's stories are suppressed by the medical community, big Pharma and the American press.

"There is a total refusal to have the discussion and derision towards anyone who tries."

The facts didn't seem to matter at the *Times*. The damage being done to a generation of children isn't their concern, either. Supporting the make-believe science coming out of the CDC was all they cared about.

I asked Dr. Haley about the accuracy of the account of the *Times* meeting with Robert Kennedy.[19] He wrote back:

"Robert Kennedy asked me to accompany him to the *Times*, and the description in the *SPECTRUM* article is very close to how I remember the meeting. The writers were not at all interested in the published science. I would make a comment about thimerosal toxicity

. . . and they would look surprised—but they never asked for any of the stack of reports to verify what I said. Afterwards, one of the writers, a young man, whose name I don't remember, followed me out the door and downstairs, seemed interested and asked some detailed questions, but later wrote an article and did not mention any of the published science about the toxicity of thimerosal. I lost a lot of respect for the *New York Times* that day and felt quite sorry for Robert Kennedy, who was just asking for a logical look at the autism/vaccine issue. The *Times* did the opposite and wrote totally supporting the CDC line that their experts had eliminated vaccines as being involved."

Despite the initial interest by the media, the issue of vaccines and a link to autism faded from investigative journalism. It was much easier to simply cite the official denials. The press retreated to the pat claim that "studies show no link" between vaccines and the new phenomenon of autism. Kirby's work didn't lead to more investigation by the media. The use of toxic mercury in vaccines continued to be considered acceptable and safe. The fact that it was still present in the majority of flu vaccine wasn't of interest to the mainstream media.

March 22, 2010, in Robert Kennedy, Jr.'s broadcast of his show, *Ring of Fire*, he interviewed Dr. Haley.[20] The focus of their talk was a possible bribery scandal involving the Centers for Disease Control and a Danish vaccine researcher.

Kennedy: "Dr. Poul Thorsen, who is the principal author of the leading study that CDC . . . has cited for eight years as the proof positive that there is no connection between the autism epidemic and the mercury-laced vaccines . . . the principal author of that study . . . has now vanished, apparently having stolen millions of dollars of funds that he received from the taxpayers through the CDC, that he had supposedly spent on research. But he has taken those funds and disappeared."

Haley expressed his outrage at the vaccine-safety research that Thorsen had conducted.

Haley: "The data and the manipulation of the data in those studies, and results, the conclusions of those studies were ridiculous. For example, they claimed that they took thimerosal out of vaccines in Denmark... thimerosal is a very potent neurotoxin . . . the autism rate went up. And according to a graph, it went up almost twentyfold. That's equivalent to saying that you took the alcohol away from the person that was drinking, and they got drunker. It's just preposterous.

"If you look at the funding and the projects and the papers . . . Poul Thorsen did while he was at Emory, all his research was designed to find something other than the vaccines that could possibly cause autism. . . . The CDC is funding someone to cover their back door. . . . It's a waste of taxpayer dollars.

"Instead of going and finding what the real cause is by looking at these kids biochemically, they hired a person who's a psychiatrist. Biological research isn't the strong suit of people with degrees in psychiatry."

Kennedy asked Haley how much independent research on mercury-laced vaccines there was out there.

Haley: "There's lots of it. Almost all the research . . . on the biochemical or physiological level indicates it's mercury toxic. And plus the logic is there. We now know it's not genetic. They spent, at the behest of the CDC and the Institute of Medicine 2004 committee, they've spent scores of millions of dollars to look for the genetic cause of autism—and there just couldn't possibly have been a genetic cause for this epidemic."

The two major news sources that had published Kennedy's "Deadly Immunity," *Salon.com* and *Rolling Stone,* came under pressure, and, in 2011, *Salon.com* retracted the publication.[21] *CBS Money Watch* reported on Jan. 22, 2011 that *Rolling Stone* had done the same, and CBS called the claim that vaccines were linked to autism "utter garbage," but by May, 2011, *Rolling Stone* reposted Kennedy's story.[22]

When the story was reposted in *Rolling Stone*, this was added:

"Editor's Note: The link to this much-debated story by Robert F. Kennedy, Jr. was inadvertently broken during our redesign in the spring of 2010. (We did not remove the story from the site, as some have incorrectly alleged, nor ever contemplated doing so.) The link to the original story is now restored, including the corrections we posted at the time and the subsequent editorial we published about the ensuing controversy."

In 2005, David Kirby and Robert Kennedy, Jr. sounded an alarm all over in the media. They raised serious concerns about the use of a known neurotoxin in children's vaccines. The questions they asked were never answered.

# CHAPTER SIX
# GENERATION RESCUE

*"We don't want to be too narrow-minded and say it's only the vaccines, and ignore other potential problems."*

—Dr. Jim Sears, *The Doctors*, May 7, 2009

One of the formidable voices out there calling attention to the epidemic of autism and the link to vaccines has been a parent organization called Generation Rescue, dedicated to recovering children with autism.

JB Handley, founder of Generation Rescue, put it this way:

"No parent plans to be an autism activist—it just happens. In my case, watching my middle son disappear after too many vaccines and rounds of antibiotics spurred me into action. You won't make a lot of friends at the CDC or the American Academy of Pediatrics saying the things I say publicly, but I really don't care. The majority of autism parents agree with me: Something about our shot schedule is sending our kids into autism. I'm proud to play a small role in helping children recover, and, hopefully, sooner than later, I can help put an end to this man-made madness."[1]

In 2008, Jenny McCarthy joined Handley at Generation Rescue. McCarthy is a well-known public figure, often blamed for promoting the controversial claim that vaccines can cause autism. She's written a number of books on the subject that have been

*New York Times* best sellers: *Louder Than Words: A Mother's Journey in Healing Autism; Mother Warriors: A Nation of Parents Healing Autism Against All Odds;* and *Healing and Preventing Autism,* co-written with Dr. Jerry Kartzinel.

On April 2, 2008, International Autism Awareness Day, McCarthy was a guest on CNN's *Larry King Live,* discussing her book *Louder Than Words.*[2] She talked about the importance of designating April 2 for autism. "It's a global epidemic, and it's not going to get any better until change is implemented." King asked McCarthy about her son, and she said that just before the age of three, her son, Evan, began having life-threatening seizures and subsequently was diagnosed with autism. Because of her research on the Internet, she was able to connect with an organization called Defeat Autism Now. Their doctors provided her with a protocol to recover her son.

As she often has done, at this point in the interview, McCarthy insisted, "I'm not, nor is the autism community, anti-vaccine. We're anti-toxin, and we're anti-schedule." She said that many parents she knows are treating their children from vaccine injury, and they're getting better.

McCarthy cited the dramatic increase in the vaccine schedule from ten vaccines in 1983 to thirty-six shots by 2008 and the coincidental explosion in the autism rate and the countless parents who say it was the vaccines.

The medical community has closed its eyes to what countless parents have reported, in her view. "I believe that parents' anecdotal information is science-based information. And when the entire world is screaming the same thing, 'Doctor, I came home, he had a fever, he stopped speaking, and then became autistic.' . . . it's time to start listening to that."

McCarthy continued, explaining how, because of biomedical treatments, Evan was now recovered from his autism and no longer qualifies for services, although he still has seizures and gut issues. She said that a child can't be cured of a vaccine injury but that they can get better and regain lost skills.

Jay Gordon, MD, was also on the show. He was an impressive addition to the broadcast, being a nationally known pediatrician, member of the American Academy of Pediatrics, and Assistant Professor of Pediatrics at UCLA Medical School.

Gordon was hesitant about blaming every case of autism on vaccines, but he was clear that there was a link. He said there many environmental triggers possible, "but vaccines do contribute."

McCarthy and then boyfriend Jim Carrey appeared on *Larry King Live* on April 3, 2009. McCarthy started out saying that when her son Evan was diagnosed with autism, to find any information she had to go to the Internet, where she learned about the biomedical treatments that can actually improve the health of kids with autism.

Jim Carrey described what Evan was like when he first met Jenny McCarthy. He said the boy displayed a lot of the signs of classic autism, including alienation from his surroundings and lack of affection. This all changed when McCarthy started biomedical treatments—things like a GFCF diet. He said Evan is now "a fully functioning person."

Carrey added, "I believe that autism, in my heart, is preventable and treatable."

Jenny McCarthy announced that Evan has recovered for autism and that there are thousands of other children who are doing the same. She said she had asked the doctors from the AAP to meet with the specialists who are recovering these children, but they have refused to do that.

According to Jim Carrey, the actions of the AAP made no sense. He said that he couldn't understand why they wouldn't want to learn how to help autistic kids get better.

Despite the fact that Jenny McCarthy is universally labeled as "anti-vaccine," both Carrey and McCarthy were adamant that they were not opposed to vaccinating children. Carrey said, "We're not saying, 'Don't vaccinate.' That's one thing we want to get really clear."

Next the discussion turned to the increase in the vaccine schedule after 1989. Carrey questioned the sudden need for so many new vaccines, and McCarthy said it was "greed."

They went on to tell parents to educate themselves. Carrey made a critical point when he said, "I don't think we can afford to assume that the people who are charged with our public health any longer have our best interest at heart all the time."

McCarthy said that vaccine injury isn't just about autism. Her son also developed seizures at the same time as his autism.

Larry King cited the new book by Jenny McCarthy and Jerry Kartzinel, MD, *Healing and Preventing Autism*. He asked why doctors and organizations wouldn't want to know about how to help kids disabled with autism, and Carrey immediately started talking about the money ties between the medical community and the vaccine makers.

"Vaccines are the largest growing division of the pharmaceutical industry. Thirteen billion dollars."

In part two of the Larry King broadcast, Jim Carrey and Jenny McCarthy were joined by McCarthy's co-author, Jerry Kartzinel, MD, who is also the father of an autistic son, along with JB Handley, founder of Generation Rescue.

Larry King addressed the issue of vaccines as the cause of autism. He said that two months earlier, the federal vaccine court, in three test cases representing 5,000 cases, ruled that neither vaccines containing the mercury-based vaccine preservative thimerosal nor the live virus MMR vaccine could cause autism.

According to Handley, this didn't prove anything. "Our kids get thirty-six vaccines. The MMR is two of the thirty-six shots. Before their first MMR vaccine, they get twenty-three other vaccines."

Jenny McCarthy then held up a chart showing the CCD vaccine schedule. Handley continued, "Saying that the MMR or that vaccines do not cause autism because of this one vaccine, is like having a plane crash, suspecting mechanical failure, looking at one wing, saying that one wing is safe, therefore, the whole plane is safe."

Next, Larry King asked Dr. Kartzinel about his training in autism and the fact that his son has the disorder. Kartzinel told him that during his years in medical school he'd only seen one autistic child. King asked him if there's been a real increase in autism, and he responded, "I'm definitely saying it's increased." Kartzinel blamed it on exposure to toxins—including those in our vaccines. He talked about how dangerous it is to expose pregnant women to the mercury in the flu shot. "The flu vaccine has never been shown to be safe for fetuses, and yet we're going ahead and asking our women to take that."

JB Handley went on to talk about the troubling high infant-mortality rate in this country. His claimed that the countries with smaller vaccine schedule didn't have the number of infants dying that we do and that they also don't have the autism rates that we do. Handley cited other First World countries that refused to add vaccines like chicken pox and rotavirus.

When he was asked what his position on all these controversial topics had done to his standing in the medical community, Kartzinel said it had definitely made him an outcast. He told King that other pediatricians weren't interested in learning about the biomedical treatments or the link to vaccines.

Next Dr. Kartzinel held up a recent copy of *Pediatrics*, the official journal of the American Academy of Pediatrics, and cited a survey which he said showed, "Doctors do not want to take care of autistic children. They don't want to learn about them."

Recognizing the dedication that Kartzinel brought to this issue, King asked him about the impact of autism on him personally.

Kartzinel said that his son's regression after the MMR vaccine changed the way he practiced pediatric medicine. He learned how to effectively treat his autistic patients. In his words, "It's my whole practice. It's everything that I do."

King wanted the specifics about how vaccines cause autism, and Handley told him that they cause brain damage. For Handley, this explained why the numbers went from one in 10,000, forty years ago, to one in a hundred today.

King brought up the possibility that because of discussions like the one they were having, parents might decide not to vaccinate. For McCarthy, it didn't matter. If vaccines were safer, parents would vaccinate.

Jenny McCarthy's appearance on Larry King and other places has not gone unnoticed. She continues to be demonized by the media and the medical community for spreading the idea that vaccines cause autism and telling parents not to vaccinate.

Incredibly, when stories denounce her as "anti-vaccine" and "an ex-Playboy bunny," they conveniently forget to mention the medical experts backing her up. The public isn't told that she co-authored the book *Healing and Preventing Autism* with Dr. Kartzinel.

Nothing is said about the foreword to her 2007 book, *Louder Than Words—A Mother's Journey in Healing Autism*. It was written by David Feinberg, MD, chief executive officer of the UCLA Hospital System and associate vice chancellor.

It would be very difficult to dismiss McCarthy's claims if Drs. Feinberg, Kartzinel, and Gordon were included in the reporting. That's probably why we never get to hear about them.

The media is very selective about who they blame for parents linking vaccines to autism. All the research showing vaccines can harm us and the experts who dispute the safety claims are neatly ignored. Still, the medical community can't avoid talking about the controversy that just won't go away.

On Dec 3, 2008, the popular show *The Doctors* began with Dr. Travis Stork telling the audience about measles outbreaks and "pockets of children where there are communities where parents are choosing not to vaccinate their kids."[3]

Dr. Jim Sears continued the discussion, citing the controversy over the MMR and autism. "Maybe ten years ago, this thing with autism came up, but that's really seemed to have settled down a lot. Most of the evidence linking measles vaccine with autism has kind of settled down. And most of the doctors and scientists agree that it probably isn't the major cause."

That was an incredible comment. A well-known medical expert had acknowledged that there was a link between the MMR vaccine and autism on a nationally seen television show. He downplayed the significance of his admission by saying that "it probably isn't the major cause," but the audience was left with the disturbing truth that, according to Dr. Sears, the MMR vaccine could cause autism.

Next, Sears talked about the dangers associated with having measles and why the vaccine is so important. The audience was left to consider that the vaccine that is said to prevent measles may also lead to autism.

To provide a balance in the show, Barbara Loe Fisher was shown sitting in the audience. Dr. Stork asked her about "the message we're sending to moms, because if they don't vaccinate, we could have a measles outbreak, and it could become an epidemic where like years ago, four million people are getting the measles."

Fisher talked about how back in 1980, she had taken her two-and-a-half-year-old in for his DPT vaccine. Within hours, he had a violent reaction, including seizures and unconsciousness. She said he was later diagnosed with minor brain damage and learning disabilities.

As far as the threat of measles outbreaks was concerned, Fisher said, "A hundred and thirty-one cases of measles out of three hundred million people is not an epidemic. We have a ninety-eight percent vaccination rate."

Fisher, looking very intense, said, "We have more than tripled the number of doses of vaccines we're giving our children in the last quarter century. At the same time, we have seen children become disabled and chronically ill." She listed the exploding rates of autism, asthma, learning disabilities, and diabetes among kids in America, and asked why this highly vaccinated population is so sick and disabled.

After Barbara Loe Fisher's brief air time, the doctors took turns informing the audience about the mechanics of vaccination—how a vaccine works.

Next, there was another guest on stage, introduced as Julia, who raised serious concerns about the one-size-fits-all vaccination schedule in the US. She talked about her three children. Her oldest had been vaccinated with "a huge amount of mercury," and he received the MMR. Julia described what happened to him: loss of language and social skills and loss of bowel control. The reaction began only a few hours after receiving his vaccines. He was diagnosed with autism. His mother referred to him as her "sacrificial lamb."

At this point, Julia made her position on vaccine clear. She said that her first child had gotten burned. "Don't ask me to line up my other two children to get burned again. What kind of parent would I be?" It's easy to imagine the reaction in the minds of the mothers in the audience and the ones watching the broadcast. There must have been lots of questions: What if this happened to my child? How could anyone blame her for not vaccinating? Who can I trust?

Just the fact that Julia appeared on *The Doctors* gave her a lot of credibility. There must be something to what she's saying. Her child's experience sounded a lot like what happened to Barbara Loe Fisher's son.

The conversation then turned to a discussion of the vaccination requirement for children to attend school. Julia asked about what happens to kids where there is a familial history of vaccine reaction. Dr. Sears said that he had families like this in his practice and that he was against mandatory vaccines. "I think somebody should have the right to say, 'No.'"

Sears brought up autism, saying that some studies show no link and that others show a possible link. He'd looked at the issue for the last several years, coming to the conclusion that "it probably isn't just the vaccines."

Whether the audience recognized it or not, that was an shocking admission: "It probably isn't just the vaccines." Vaccines were in no way supposed to be connected to autism. Here a doctor is telling parents there really is a connection. Vaccinate at your own risk. And, for Dr. Sears, this was a very courageous step. Speaking out against one of the strongest tenets in modern medicine must have had some repercussions.

Then Julia brought up the need for a comparison study of vaccinated and unvaccinated children. "No one is doing that study. That study needs to be done." Sears backed her up. He said, "One size does not fit all."

Things got even more amazing on this broadcast. Stork made a statement rarely heard from a doctor. He said, "I tell you. I tend to agree with Dr. Sears that, hey, if you're a mom and you're educated, and you don't want your kids to be vaccinated, you should have that choice—if you're making an informed decision—in my opinion."

Immediately following Dr. Stork's comment, a doctor in the audience returned to the claim that herd immunity is vital. Besides, vaccines today are much improved over vaccines from thirty years ago. Julia wasn't buying his assurances. She said she didn't trust the vaccine makers. Their interest is financial. That comment was followed by applause from the audience.

Barbara Loe Fisher was shown calling for informed consent. She said it was one of the central principles of medicine. Parents should have the right to choose.

As Fisher spoke, faces in the audience were shown. They were women, and they looked concerned. The people on this show admitted that vaccines carry risks—including autism. The possibility of a child developing autism from vaccination was real.

Other topics were covered during the show. Dr. Stork asked Fisher if we've traded infectious for chronic illness. Stork credited vaccine with increasing life expectancy. Gesturing toward Julia, he pointed out that regardless of the "terrible tragedy" she experienced, vaccines do save lives.

Stork ended the show announcing, "The overwhelming majority of pediatricians in this country strongly support vaccination."

Anyone paying close attention during this show had to understand that these experts weren't denying a link, but they were saying it's worth it to take the risk. Viewers were left with the frightening realization that vaccination was a gamble.

To their credit, *The Doctors* covered this topic again the following year.

On May 7, 2009, Jenny McCarthy was on *The Doctors* to discuss vaccines and autism.[4] This should have raised questions. Why would a network broadcast with leading doctors include someone who was notorious for spreading the false idea that vaccines were linked to autism?

Dr. Jim Sears started out saying that kids used to be dying of meningitis and lots of them had vaccine-preventable illnesses, but today, all the vaccines have eradicated these diseases, according to Sears. He didn't want parents to stop vaccinating and cause polio to come back.

McCarthy's response was that there were too many vaccines and that there was still mercury in the flu vaccine.

Next JB Handley, seated in the audience, joined the discussion saying that we only think there are benefits from vaccinating. He cited the number of vaccines US kids get compared to other countries and how serious the US infant-mortality rate is. The countries with fewer vaccines on their schedules have lower autism rates. It was clear to Handley that was a connection here.

While Dr. Jim Sears again admitted the possibility of a link between vaccines and autism, he also seemed to try to change the focus. He stressed we shouldn't be "too narrow-minded" and say vaccines are the only cause of autism.

Dr. Travis Stork, sitting next to Sears, said that while he wanted to have "an open debate" on the issue, "vaccines are really the one thing we have looked at as causing autism."

Handley's response was immediate. He called that claim "completely bogus."

According to Handley, health officials had only looked at two vaccines on a schedule of thirty-six, and they've only studied one of the thirty-five ingredients in vaccines. Officials couldn't possibly say vaccines didn't cause autism when they had done limited research. It was like "bogus tobacco science." Handley said he was tired of experts who didn't read the studies, who told parents there was no link.

His last remarks were almost drowned out by the applause from the audience.

Dr. Stork seemed very agitated at this, and, as he gestured dramatically, he loudly proclaimed this "the biggest problem" for doctors in America. He said they're frustrated. Stork blamed Handley for "antagonizing the medical community that only wants to help those kids." He asked Handley, "Why would you do that?"

At this point in the show, lots of voices could be heard talking. Stork continued in a loud voice, "What we're trying to figure out here is how to help kids, and all you do when you yell at me on my stage, all you do is anger me."

Stork looked upset and dramatically stated, "I asked you to defend your stance, and all you did was attack me."

Incredibly, Dr. Stork seemed oblivious to what autism was doing to our children and the lives of hundreds of thousands of families—while the medical community had nothing to offer parents. Didn't parents like JB Handley have a right to be angry? So far, doctors hadn't even recognized autism as a problem.

Handley told Stork that parents were frustrated because doctors weren't listening to them. He disagreed with Stork, who said that there was no connection between vaccines and autism, saying, "It's simply not true."

The camera showed a close-up of Dr. Jerry Kartzinel, who was on the stage with Jenny McCarthy and Drs. Sears and Stork, with Dr. Stork telling viewers about all the "environmental toxins out there that could be linked to autism. Handley can't be right when he says that vaccines cause autism. He couldn't know more than "99.9 percent of pediatricians." He continued to make his case. "Vaccines have been studied."

While Sears was saying this, Handley's voice could be heard saying, "Thirty-six shots. You have to be honest about the science. We're just asking for people to be honest about what's actually been done."

This show aired in May 2009. Fourteen months earlier, the story of Hannah Poling was everywhere on the news. She was the young Georgia girl who regressed into autism after receiving nine vaccinations in a single doctor's visit. Health and Human Services recognized her vaccine injury. HHS conceded her case, and she was compensated by the government. While the media did a good job of covering the story, they tried to downplay its significance, telling the public that Hannah Poling had only "autism-like symptoms" and that she had a "rare" mitochondrial disorder that predisposed her to develop autism. At that time, there were calls for more research to find out how many other children had the same vulnerability, something that never happened.

Hannah Poling's story was groundbreaking, and, yet, it didn't even come up on this episode. Dr. Sears and Dr. Stork pretty much agreed that the science was in on vaccines, and they had no other alternative theory of causation. They both ignored that fact that according to Handley, only two vaccines out of thirty-six had actually been studied and only one vaccine ingredient out of thirty-five.

Maybe the real message from these doctors was that no one *wanted* it to be the vaccines. The consequences of this possibility would be too horrendous to imagine. Doctors like Stork tried to convince the viewers of the benefits of vaccination and assure them that all the science was in.

Generation Rescue co-founder JB Handley did more than speak out on talk shows. His organization was responsible for full-page ads in prominent newspapers that presented hundreds of thousands of readers with undeniable facts about the vaccine-autism controversy.

On May 24, 2005, an ad in *USA Today* in huge bold type read: "Autism is preventable and reversible."[5]

The message continued:

> "Today, 1 in 166 children is diagnosed with autism. It is critical that we have all the facts about this epidemic, including recent developments about autism's relationship to mercury poisoning and how the right detoxification treatment can entirely reverse the disorder.
>
> "To find out more about this life-changing news, go to *generationrescue.org*. Generation Rescue was founded for parents by parents. We are dedicated to empowering parents with the truth to help their children heal."

While the ad didn't mention the word "vaccines," it did challenge the claim by countless doctors that autism was a genetic disorder that was now so prominent only because the definition had been broadened and the medical community was doing a better job diagnosing it. It also linked toxic mercury to a disorder now called an "epidemic."

One month later, on June 8, 2005, Generation Rescue paid for a startling ad in the *New York Times.*[6] Again, the point was made that mercury can cause autism. The headline made the case: "MERCURY POISONING AND AUTISM—It isn't a coincidence."

Beneath that were two lists comparing the symptoms of autism and the symptoms of mercury poisoning, and the same seven symptoms were on each list:

"Loss of Speech, Social Withdrawal, Reduced Eye Contact, Repetitive Behaviors, Hand-flapping/Toe Walking, Temper Tantrums, Sleep Disturbances, Seizures."

Underneath that were quotes from prominent Americans: US Senator John Kerry, US Rep. Dan Burton, Robert F. Kennedy, Jr., and US Rep. Dave Weldon, all talking about the dangers of mercury.

At the bottom of the ad was a picture of David Kirby's book, *Evidence of Harm*, and two quotations about the book. One was from *the New York Times:*

"Kirby makes the unassailable point that American health agencies lagged in calculating the amount of mercury being injected into babies."

The other was from the *Financial Times:*

"Big Pharma's fortunes are tethered in part to the *Amazon.com* sales rank of *Evidence of Harm.*"

The ad also said that removing toxic mercury could reverse the symptoms of autism.

According to their websites, *USA Today* and the *New York Times* have two to three million readers. Even if a small percentage of these readers actually read the ads, lots of people were made aware that serious questions were being raised over vaccine safety. And vaccines with mercury were linked to autism.

In March 2006, a very controversial ad appeared in *USA Today* once again. In large, striking white letters on a black background, the message was clear:

"If you caused A 6,000% INCREASE IN AUTISM, wouldn't you try to cover it up?"

This was followed by a quotation from Robert F. Kennedy, Jr. "IT'S TIME FOR THE CDC TO COME CLEAN WITH THE AMERICAN PUBLIC."

The charge was straightforward:

"We believe the Centers for Disease Control (CDC) knows that the ambitious immunization schedule begun in the 1990s, nearly tripling the amount of mercury injected into our children, created an epidemic of autism in America. We are mystified that mercury remains in children's vaccines and that the CDC and American Academy of Pediatrics are fighting state laws banning mercury. Why?

"Thousands of children are recovering from autism by having the mercury removed from their bodies using the Defeat Autism Now! Protocol. Yet, the CDC doesn't investigate these stories of recovery. Why?

"We call on our elected officials, journalists, and all Americans to help us in the fight for recovery, truth, and justice for our children. As long as the CDC denies that mercury from vaccines is responsible for this epidemic, proper treatment will never be made widely available to the more than one million American children who could be treated today."

In 2007, Generation Rescue continued to get the message out to the public. This time the ad appeared in *the Orange County Register* and the *Oregonian,* two prominent papers on the West Coast.[7] The main message linked vaccines directly to autism.

On the top of the ad was a picture of a hypodermic needle and the large, dark letters with the question: "ARE WE OVER-VACCINATING OUR KIDS?" This time, there were lists of the vaccines given in 1983 and those on the schedule in 2007. In 1983, there were only ten vaccines. In 2007, there were thirty-six and vaccination beginning at birth with the hepatitis B vaccine. Bold-faced letters at the bottom of the ad answered the question, "A SURVEY OF KIDS IN CALIFORNIA AND OREGON SAYS WE MAY WELL BE."

In the ad, readers were told that Generation Rescue had hired a marketing research firm to conduct a survey of more than 17, 000 children in the states of California and Oregon. It said the results showed that vaccinated boys had a 2.5 greater chance of developing a neurological disorder than unvaccinated ones. The ad called for a national study to "explore these disturbing results."

In 2008 and 2009, additional ads appeared in *USA Today* paid for by Generation Rescue.[8]

In the 2008 ad, the focus was again the dramatic expansion of the vaccine schedule. The headline read: "ARE WE POISONING OUR KIDS IN THE NAME OF PROTECTING THEIR HEALTH?"

The next lines said:

"Green our vaccines."

"Administer them with care."

Again, there was a graphic showing the list of vaccines given in 1998 compared to more than triple the number of doses given in 2008. The vaccine ingredients mercury, aluminum, formaldehyde, ether, and antifreeze were listed in the ad.

The *USA Today* ad in 2009 alleged that the government had long known about the link between vaccines and autism.[9] Readers were told that in the vaccine-injury case of Bailey Banks, a federal vaccine court had ruled that vaccination led to autism. Just as in the case of Hannah Poling, announced a year earlier, the government would compensate the family.

"Small victories for these children, but what about the hundreds of thousands of other families struggling with autism? Who and what can they believe in this continuing vaccine-autism controversy?

"Congress, at the urging of the pharmaceutical industry, created the mysterious Vaccine Court in1986, which has not only protected vaccine makers from liability but also led to a tripling in the number of vaccines given to our children.

"Why does the Vaccine Court exist? Why are the rulings in favor of the children being suppressed? Where is the justice for these parents?"

Most of the people reading what appeared in *USA Today* in 2009 had probably never heard about the existence of a "Vaccine Court." For many of them, it might have been the first time they had ever considered that vaccines could have serious side effects. With all the news coverage on afternoon talk shows, mainstream news, and national newspapers, the link between vaccines and autism was now firmly in the public's consciousness.

The Generation Rescue ads weren't the only things getting the public's attention by 2009. In March 2009, the National Vaccine Information Center and *Mercola.com* sponsored a fifteen-second message on the CBS Jumbotron on Times Square in New York.[10]

The message was simple:

"Vaccines: Know the risks.

"Vaccination, Your Health. Your Family. Your Choice."

On April 13, 2011, the president of the American Academy of Pediatrics contacted CBS to pressure them into removing the Jumbotron message.[11] Barbara Loe Fisher, the head of the NVIC, put out a recorded statement on the actions of the AAP. She also said that the AAP had been on the receiving end of undisclosed donations from the pharmaceutical industry.

In November 2011, NVIC sponsored ads on Delta Airline flights about preventing the flu. The video was about three minutes long, and Barbara Loe Fisher spoke. She pointed out the fact that eighty percent of the time when you get the symptoms of the flu—the cough, fever, runny nose, body aches—you don't have type A or type B influenza.

The video recommended washing hands, covering your month, drinking fluids, getting plenty of sleep, and taking vitamins as ways of preventing the flu. Next, the issue of getting a flu vaccine was addressed, and viewers were told to "research the types of flu vaccines your doctor may recommend."

The video message urged people to study the information that comes with the flu shot, especially about "who should and who shouldn't get the vaccine." There was nothing anti-vaccine about this video. It simply urged people to be informed about a medical product. Nevertheless, the American Academy of Pediatrics spoke out against the ad. In a *Forbe*s story on November 7, 2011, the AAP said that the Delta Airline ad "urges viewers to become informed about influenza and how to stay well during the flu season without resorting to the influenza vaccine."[12] This, despite the fact that nothing in the message told people not to get the vaccine.

In December 2011, the NVIC vaccine-safety message was again up in Times Square.[13] The ad was fifteen seconds in length and appeared twice an hour on the megatron starting on December 16. It was also up for the huge News Year's Eve celebration in New York.

Those who didn't accept that a one-size-fits-all vaccination schedule is safe for everyone were making their voices heard. The very public statements made by Generation Rescue and the National Vaccine Information Center were brief and to the point: parents need to worry that the one-size-fits-all vaccination schedule simply doesn't fit.

# CHAPTER SEVEN
# THE GREATER GOOD

*"Even were such a link proved definitively, all that matters is that its victims number significantly fewer than those of the diseases vaccinations are designed to prevent."*

—*New York Times* review of *The Greater Good*, Nov. 17, 2011

In 2011, a stunning film was released that would once again tie autism to vaccine injury. The movie was called *The Greater Good*, produced by Leslie Manookian, Kendall Nelson, and Chris Pilaro.[1] As its title implies, it dealt with the obvious reality that when we vaccinate our children, we also accept the risks in order to provide herd immunity for all children.

*The Greater Good* showed us three stories of vaccine injury. One involved a teenage girl damaged by the cervical-cancer vaccine Gardasil, another was about a baby who died of SIDS following vaccination, and finally a boy who became autistic after being vaccinated.

Viewers were told about Jordan King, age eleven, of Portland, Oregon, who regressed into autism following routine vaccinations and was one of the test cases for the Autism Omnibus Proceedings. His case was ultimately rejected by a special master in Vaccine Court.

The film shows the parents in their home.

MyLinda King, Jordan's mother: "As a baby, Jordan was just a typical baby. He met his milestones and was ahead of the curve on a few of them, very social, had great eye contract. Everybody just said what a great little guy he was. We just noticed over a few months that he no longer spoke. He started walking on his toes all the time and flapping his hands when he would get excited or over-stimulated."

In the next scene, Jordan's parents reflect as they look over his baby pictures. MyLinda King points to one photo and says, "That's one of the first pictures where you can see something is wrong."

Jordan's dad, Fred King, says, "His eyes weren't as lively."

Mother: "I can't explain it, but it was like the sparkle was gone. He looked sad all the time."

MyLinda King describes taking Jordan to the pediatrician. "She just said, 'Oh, he's autistic. That's how it goes sometimes. They're born that way.' But we felt like there was something medically going on with him, so we took him to this doctor, and he said, 'The first thing I want to do is check him for heavy metals.'"

Jordan's test results showed the heavy-metal burden he had. "The mercury was off the end of the page. I sort of freaked out. I thought, he's mercury poisoned. Where did that mercury come from?"

Jordan's dad describes their search for answers. "We tested the paint. We tested the air. I had the sawdust in my basement shop tested to see, is there mercury in that? When we talked to Dr. Green about it and told him what we were doing, he said, 'You don't have to look for where the mercury's coming from. We know where it's coming from. It's in the vaccines that Jordan's been getting.'"

The next scene shows Jordan and his mother at his doctor's office. In a voiceover, family practitioner Dr. John Green III describes his practice since he started in medicine back in 1975. "I saw one child with autism in the eighties, one child with autism in the early nineties, and, then, in the late nineties, I was literally flooded with patients. I've evaluated and treated now approximately twenty-one hundred patients with autism."

MyLinda and the doctor discuss how Jordan gets his needs met, since he's not able to speak. She's shown saying, "When he wants to eat a hot meal, he'll bring me a spatula and a hot-pad."

Dr. Green continues to explain what the mercury in his vaccines did to Jordan. "Jordan received mercury far exceeding EPA safety guidelines. We know that mercury causes neurotoxicity. There's no controversy about that. Does it cause autism? It contributes to the damages that lead to autism. Jordan was not born with autism. He was a normal child. He was injured by vaccinations, and the injuries led to his autism."

The next scene in the film shows Lawrence Palevsky, MD, who says, "Certainly this is a controversial point in the medical field because the conventional medical community has basically stated that there is no link between mercury and autism."

Vaccine developer Dr. Paul Offit follows, "The science has been very clear on this. We have six studies showing mercury-containing vaccines don't cause autism. And although there can be slight flaws, I think, in any of those studies, once you have negative study after negative study after negative study, I think you can say with comfort that a truth has emerged."

Offit's comment is immediately challenged by Barbara Loe Fisher, head of the National Vaccine Information Center, a national charitable, non-profit educational organization founded in 1982. Fisher states simply, "Almost all vaccine studies are epidemiological studies, which means that large groups of people are compared to each other. There has been very little bench science that is looking at what happens at the molecular and cellular level in the body. We really need to do both kinds of study in order to understand what really happens."

The film goes back to covering Dr. Green. "The research is incomplete, and the certainty that's foisted on us by vaccine authorities is not scientific."

*The Greater Good* then highlights a quotation from 1999: "The American Academy of Pediatrics and vaccine manufacturers agreed that thimerosal should be reduced or eliminated in vaccines as a precautionary measure."

Dr. Palevsky appears saying, "Since 1999, the amount of mercury has been reduced in vaccinations, but thimerosal is still present in some vaccines. And it's pretty clear from the scientific evidence that any form of mercury in the body is toxic and that it can cause damage."

Then a graphic image reads, "The CDC recommends a flu shot each year for every child and adult." The next image says, "Most flu shots contain mercury."

Following this, the scene shows Dr. Green, Jordan, and Jordan's mother at the end of his doctor visit. MyLinda Jordan says, "We're still hoping that he can learn to articulate a few words because I think he's becoming aware that he can't talk. I think that's finally frustrating him. . . . Sometimes he'll get up in my mouth and just watch me talk like, how do you do that?"

Then, there's a close-up of Dr. Green. "The bottom line is, there are great differences between children. We make assumptions that every child has a similar level of tolerance, which is clearly not the case. There is a study looking at children's hair for mercury showing autistic children excreting much less mercury compared to other children. Clearly there's some inability to get rid of the toxics, so they're much more susceptible."

Later in the film, Jordan and his mother are shown playing with toys on the floor. She describes him. "I would say he acts like your average maybe three- or four-year-old. It's kind of like having a toddler for eleven years. People will email me and say, 'It's such a blessing to have a child with autism. We're so lucky. We learn so much from our son. He's an angel. He isn't corrupted by the world.'"

MyLinda King can't understand that reaction. Jordan is shown on the floor, making sounds softly as she says, "Having a kid with autism is really hard, and it's not what the kid would have wanted for himself. It obviously makes you stronger and tougher, but it's not a blessing. It's pretty hard."

MyLinda continues while the film shows a crowd of parents at an outdoor meeting.

"Almost eight years ago, we were at an autism rally, and we started to talk to other people; everybody had the same story about the mercury toxicity. And this one parent, George Meade, decided to go ahead with this class action, and we decided to join him in that. Jordan and William Meade were two of the test cases that were chosen to represent the lawsuit."

A slide then shows the words, "Jordan King was one of 5,600 cases in the omnibus autism proceedings that examined the link between autism and vaccines."

*The Greater Good* presents an additional medical expert here with serious concerns about vaccine safety. Robert Sears, MD, appears next and says, "Where the research is going on this is to try to identify which children have some sort of genetic risk or some sort of predisposition to having a severe vaccine reaction."

MyLinda King: "The first thing we learned is you can't sue the drug company that made the vaccine. Our lawyer explained to us that there was this court set up specifically to address all the vaccine injuries."

Next, the vaccine-injury lawyers and Barbara Loe Fisher describe the establishment of a special compensation program that has paid out billions for vaccine injuries, supported by a tax paid on each vaccine that's given in the US. A slide reads, "Vaccine makers . . . are poised to generate $21.5 billion in annual sales . . ."

Fisher continues, "We face a future where, presumably, you could have thirty, forty, fifty different vaccines recommended for universal use, mandated, and absolutely no accountability. You have a prescription for disaster when you don't have anybody accountable in a court of law for what happens when vaccines go wrong."

Viewers next see three of the injury lawyers in a restaurant discussing how the Vaccine Injury Compensation Program works. "It just amazes me what the government does to protect the integrity of vaccines. It can be anything but the vaccine. They feel as though their job is to keep immunization rates up. If you legitimize vaccine claims, then you're saying, 'Yeah, there are vaccine injuries.' And they can never say that."

They describe the motives of the government as "well-meaning" and "profitable for the pharmaceuticals."

At one point in the film, while cartoon images of children passing by on a conveyor belt appear, in a voiceover, Palevsky speaks. "The vaccine program is one-size-fits-all. Every child is the same. Every child needs to be vaccinated, regardless of their family history or their medical background. What we don't know is what is sitting in their genetics that's potentially going to express itself or not express itself for a child to develop certain chronic illnesses."

Later, Palevsky is shown with a mother and a little boy in his office while his voiceover can be heard: "When I trained in the 1980s, one of the things that my mentors taught me was always listen to the mother. The mother knows the child. I see a lot of children whose parents come to me knowing that the child was damaged by vaccines. That's anecdotal. There's no study there. We need to do a proper scientific study comparing the health outcomes of children who are vaccinated to health outcomes of children who are not vaccinated."

Immediately, Dr. Bob Sears appears speaking, as if to complete the thought, saying, "Until we have that placebo-controlled unvaccinated group compared to a large vaccinated group, there's always going to be doubts in parents' minds."

It is very difficult to watch these scenes and not worry that there might be something potentially harmful in a mandated schedule.

The trailer for *The Greater Good* shows Barbara Loe Fisher saying, "In the last three decades, the number of doses of vaccines have more than tripled."

Listeners hear, "The majority of vaccine research is paid for by the vaccine manufacturers themselves."

It's hard to listen to experts telling viewers that vaccinations do carry risks and you have no guarantee that your child won't be affected. *The Greater Good* also presented the stories of two other children. Gabi Swank, fifteen, from Wichita, KS, was left with seizures, vasculitis, and chronic illness following the Gardasil vaccine for cervical cancer. Stephanie Christner, MD, of Tulsa, OK, lost her five-month-old daughter to SIDS and then found studies that documented vaccine injuries published in major medical journals going back decades.

Jordan King's mother makes the point, "I wish they would stop saying that we're anti-vaccine. I think that's just a way of labeling us that makes it easy for people to dismiss us." According to King, "There's no middle ground. Either you accept vaccines as safe, or you don't. Either we have to do it the way we've been doing it, or you don't do it at all."

In the following segment, a news report from ABC7 says, "A landmark court ruling doesn't mince words—vaccines do not cause autism. The theory of vaccine-related causation, the court ruled, is scientifically unsupportable. This is a case where the evidence is so one-sided . . ."

Vaccine court lawyer Kevin Conway: "It was a case unlike any other. It was very, very public. The news media was very, very much involved, and because of all the publicity, the fear on behalf of the government was great that vaccines were going to be considered unsafe."

MyLinda King: "The government's lawyers were treating our whole side as if we ignore science and we were not rational people.

The only people I know of who've received awards left the word 'autism' out of the equation. Anything but the 'A' word. Somehow this autism-vaccine thing became so political and so explosive." As King says this, a slide shows the words, "Brain Injuries Caused by Vaccines. US Government Paid 1,322 Claims."

King: "I just want everyone to lay down their arms, and let's figure out what is making them so sick."

Later in the film, the focus is again on Jordan King. Jordan and his dad are shown at the end of a bike ride. The voiceover is by Fred King. "Overall, the one feeling I have is low-level, constant anxiety. You have to constantly monitor what other people think about what's going on. Sometimes I almost want to wear a T-shirt, 'I have autism, I can't talk,' or something like that."

MyLinda King continues the narration. "There have been several incidences here in Portland with autistic teenagers and adults getting tasered by police. The police will yell at you to stop or turn around because you're acting weird so that they think you're on drugs. We're not spring chickens. He's obviously going to outlive us. We're hoping that by the time he's an adult, there's some kind of group home that evolves, because those kids are coming down the pike. About ten years from now, there's going to be a lot of autistic people out there walking the streets."

It's hard to imagine anyone not being concerned after viewing this film. The question was, of course, "How would the media report on this?" Would all the experts and all the injured kids presented in *The Greater Good* somehow be ignored, explained away, or challenged?

The *Wall Street Journal* covered *The Greater Good* on April 3, 2011, admitting at the beginning of the story that this movie "could intensify debate around the potential dangers of vaccines."[2] The piece went on to note that it's wrong to classify anyone who raises questions about vaccines as "anti-vaccine." The producer and co-director Chris Pilaro was quoted saying, "The media has said that if you question the current status quo, you are anti-vaccine. But all of the doctors, researchers, and scientists in our film are pro-vaccine. You should not be considered anti-vaccine to question the safety of any pharmaceutical product."

*The Greater Good* continued to get mainstream media attention. On October 13, 2011, a week before its theatrical release in Los Angeles, the *LA Weekly* covered the film.[3] Veronika Ferdman wrote that the girl, Gabi Swank, the teenager injured by Gardasil, was "particularly heartbreaking." Ferdman noted that controversy was at the heart of this. "Though there are pro-vaccine interviewees, this film has a clear agenda in encouraging skepticism toward vaccination. Producers/directors Nelson and Pilaro beg for public awareness—something that the drug companies who profit from developing and selling the vaccines are resolutely against. (That most vaccine research is funded by the vaccine manufacturers themselves is, the filmmakers convincingly argue, as effective as a fox minding the chicken coop.)"

The next day, October 14, 2011, *the Los Angeles Times* published their review of the movie.[4] Gary Goldstein wrote about the credibility of *The Greater Good*. "An articulate array of doctors, scientists and public health officials weigh in on both sides of the debate. Some cite that vaccines, often government mandated, are sound and necessary for 'the greater good,' while others demand further research, safety, and education to help parents—and everyone else—to make more informed choices before rushing to immunize.

"Either way, the film proves an effective eye-opener."

On October 16, 2011, *Variety* published a review of the film by John Anderson.[5] Anderson began by attacking the premise of the film: "Claiming the moral high ground while swimming in ethical contradictions, *The Greater Good* addresses the hot-button issue of childhood immunizations, tackling the topic in a manner that will have only one immediate outcome: Fewer kids will be vaccinated."

What seemed to bother Anderson about the film was that although it included proponents on both sides of the issue, the stories of vaccine injury would frighten parents into not vaccinating. Anderson cited the three cases discussed in the film: "A former high school cheerleader in Wichita, Kansas, who suffered disabling strokes after taking Gardasil; a young boy in Portland, Oregon, who developed autism caused by the heavy metals in his vaccines; and the parents of a baby girl whose death was linked to infancy's ordinarily routine bombardment of shots," and immediately he added, "None of these calamities should have happened." According to Anderson, the film's "very sympathetic victims" are part of its "stealthy" propaganda we need to balance the "downside" with the benefits of vaccination.

The downside here included death, chronic illness and lifelong dependency.

Anderson seemed untroubled that nothing is being done to make sure there aren't more calamities like the three highlighted in the film. He failed to note the fact that vaccine makers have no liability for their products or that a number of experts were willing to challenge the blanket safety claims of mainstream medicine and public health officials. Just asking questions and citing the damage was too risky.

The film's theatrical release took place in New York in November 2011. The *New York Times* reviewed the film in the article, "The Fight Over Vaccines and Autism, Continued" by Jeannette Catsoulis on November 17, 2011.[6]

It was not kind to those who were living with vaccine-injured children. There was no acknowledgement of Jordan King's regression into autism after vaccination or the death of Stephanie Christner's baby because of SIDS, also after routine vaccination. Instead, the *New York Times* emphasized the benefits of vaccines and left readers with the chilling proposal that even if vaccines do cause autism, all that matters is that there are more children who were saved from disease than those who developed autism.

"If the title of your documentary is *The Greater Good,* shouldn't you at least define what that is? Apparently not, as this emotionally manipulative, heavily partial look at the purported link between autism and childhood immunization would much rather wallow in the distress of specific families than engage with the needs of the population at large."

The *Times* made a stunning concession in the review that recognized these children as just collateral damage. Catsoulis wrote, "While the film acknowledges that science has so far been consistent in its refutation of a vaccine-autism link, it fails to point out that even were such a link proved definitively, all that matters is that its victims number significantly fewer than those of the diseases vaccinations are designed to prevent." She called this the "fundamental flaw" in the movie. "A cost-benefit analysis is completely ignored," and she reminded readers of the "horrors of measles, mumps, and chickenpox."

Catsoulis called the evidence against vaccines to be "anecdotal and blatant grandstanding."

Other news reports included the *Idaho Mountain Express* in Ketchum, Idaho, on March 16, 2012, which was local coverage for the film's producer, Leslie Manookian.[7] Reporter Jennifer Tuohy called the subject of the film, "the thorny issue of childhood immunizations." When Manookian was asked if vaccine makers put profit ahead of safety when it comes to making vaccines, she answered that the CEO of a vaccines company is supposed to "maximize shareholder profit." That's how they keep their jobs.

Manookian questioned why we have all the additional vaccines like flu shots, chicken pox and the hepatitis B vaccine given at birth although there is little chance of a baby getting the disease.

Manookian was asked about her goals in making the films. She cited the National Childhood Vaccine Injury Act of 1986 and said that this act recognized that vaccines can injure and kill some children and provides for compensation for victims. The point of the movie was to help people understand that this issue is not as black-and-white as we've been told. We have legislation that indicates vaccinations can injure and kill.

In the article, Manookian called for "a large, controlled study comparing vaccinated children and non-vaccinated children." Without this research, we have no idea how "widespread" the side effects might be. She said that this was one of the things they were calling for in this documentary. In addition, she wanted parents to have the right to choose.

Manookian described how hard it is for researchers to get funding to study vaccines for side effects. Doing a large comparison study on vaccinated and unvaccinated kids is unlikely "because most research is funded by either the pharmaceutical industry or the government, and both of those groups have a vested interest in vaccines." Furthermore, when scientists do find problems with a vaccine, they can't get funding for additional research.

In the *Express* story, Manookian cited the science that disputed the safety claims of health officials. She talked about research linking the birth dose of hepatitis B to autism and learning disabilities in boys and about the effects from the aluminum used in vaccines. There was also science linking asthma, rheumatoid arthritis, seizures, and encephalitis to vaccination. She noted that the mainstream media doesn't report on any of the research that show serious side effects from vaccines, and as long as they don't, authorities don't believe there's anything wrong. Furthermore, no one has ever looked at the effects of all the vaccines given together in the greatly expanded vaccination schedule.

Manookian was asked about informed consent when it comes to vaccinations, and her response was chilling. "I think it's almost impossible for a person to exercise informed consent on vaccinations today because adequate research hasn't been done." Despite the fact that the National Childhood Vaccine Injury Act says the parents have to be told what the risks from vaccinations are, for the most part, that doesn't happen. She said she knew of cases where doctors assured parents that "nothing is going to happen to your child." Manookian challenged that, saying vaccines have side effects, just like any drug.

The film opened in November 2011, in New York.

In *The Greater Good*, Barbara Loe Fisher made it clear that the media isn't interested in presenting both sides of the vaccine-safety debate. At one point, she is shown saying, "I do not do as much media as I did in the 1980s and 1990s. I think there has been a concerted effort in the last decade to demonize advocates like myself. In the twenty-first century, it has been much harder to get the other side of the vaccine story out by a media that's increasingly only covering one side of it."

Dr. Green described how PBS *Frontline* had handled his interview about vaccines. A segment from *Frontline* is shown in the movie, and the host of the program is heard saying, "Tonight on *Frontline, Frontline* reports on the science and politics of the bitter vaccine war." Green's account showed that this was not what *Frontline* did at all.

Green: "I spent half a day with a reporter who I felt was well-meaning, from *Frontline*. I gave a long interview. Three of my prestigious colleagues, academics, scientists, also gave interviews discussing our concerns about vaccinations. Not a word of any of our interviews appeared in the PBS *Frontline* story. Instead of a scientific discussion presenting the facts, hysterical moms were presented against white coat, Ivy League academics. I'm sick and tired of this. I see children injured every day, every day disasters in families from vaccination injuries."

I asked Leslie Manookian about her personal experiences with members of the media, and she described the unwillingness of the mainstream press to honestly report on what *The Greater Good* was about. She described the positive feedback they had gotten from the first people to see the rough cuts of the film, saying, "We had assembled an 'A' team to create the film, from a Sundance-award winning Director of Photography to a Sundance-award winning editor to an award-winning choreographer and archivist. In addition, I had spent nearly a decade researching the vaccine issue so we were all very optimistic about the chances of being accepted at the nation's top film festival."

The production team was optimistic about their prospects at the Sundance festival.

They learned that the selection committee thought *The Greater Good* was "provocative, thoughtful, beautifully made, etc., but the senior programmer's hands had been tied from above." The senior programmer and selection committee would normally have had freedom in their selection of films, but as she reported, "someone above intervened and refused to allow the film in the festival." Manookian added, "You really have to ask yourself why someone above was so afraid to screen *The Greater Good* at Sundance?"

Manookian and the other producers were critical about how the *New York Times* covered their film. They didn't believe that *Times* reporter Jeannette Catsoulis had even watched the film because her review was riddled with inaccuracies. Manookian wrote, "She condemned us for not depicting victims of polio—but we did. She charged that we omitted covering the 'forgotten horrors of measles, mumps and chickenpox'—but we did. She attributed a quote to the wrong character in the film. But the events that took place over the next day led us to believe there was something else at work, not simply a matter of pretending she watched when she hadn't.

"We read the review in the evening when it appeared online prior to running in print the next day. We were quite disappointed because it was so inaccurate and because it seemed to be more about the reviewer's dogma and belief about vaccines than about the quality of the film. But what really gave us pause was that the following day, the *New York Times* put up a note on the electronic version of the review stating that they had been contacted by the filmmakers and asked to make a correction because the review inaccurately stated that we had not addressed polio when in fact we had shown children in iron lungs and on crutches in braces suffering from polio. The truth was none of us had called the *Times*. So our PR person phoned them and asked who had called and was told it was a filmmaker. So we again checked with everyone on our team, and no one had called. So our PR person called the *Times* again and said that we had not called and asked to see a telephone log of the call, at which point the *Times* changed their story and said it was an 'anonymous reader' that had called. They then removed from their website any mention of the filmmakers having called but did at least correct the part about us not covering polio.

"However, the rest of the inaccuracies remained, and, were we to make a stink about it, they would have then simply depicted us as disgruntled filmmakers as they had already attempted to do by lying about us calling them in the first place. It was clear that this was not a review but a smear. I will never see the *New York Times* in the same light again."

Manookian described how CNN refused to cover the film, despite showing an initial interest. The network actually flew her to New York for an interview. She said, "I did the interview; then I had a terrific talk with the anchor, who was very concerned about the vaccine issue and contemplating having children soon. She was very earnest and open minded and assured me the piece would air the following night. I went to my hotel to sleep, got up early the next day, and flew home."

The producers of *The Greater Good* publicized the upcoming CNN interview on Facebook and with their partners around the world. Manookian explained, "But it didn't happen. We all tuned in to watch the day I flew home, and it never came on the show. We spoke with the show and were reassured it would air the next night. We were told the same thing all week. Friday night, it still did not air. When someone on our team called the host of the show to ask what was going on, we were told that the segment had been pulled by CNN's legal department, but when our PR person called the producer of the show, she was told that the host and the host's executive producer had pulled the piece. Who knows what truly happened? All that matters is that once again, we were not allowed to share the other side of the vaccines story with the public."

Lastly, Manookian described their experience with a woman who acquired films for Oprah Winfrey's new network, OWN. "[The woman] had seen the film and loved it. She had showed it to colleagues, and they all thought it was a great story, well made, and really important. They pitched it to OWN, and it dragged on for quite a while. Finally we got word that OWN was not going to move forward because the topic was too hot for them."

It was clear, when the subject is too controversial, when too many people are frightened of the implications, the story doesn't get covered.

# CHAPTER EIGHT
# CELEBRATING AUTISM

*"CDC is working with partners to study the prevalence of ASDs over time, so that we can find out if the number of children with these disorders is rising, dropping, or staying the same."*

—From the current website of the Centers for Disease Control and Prevention

Every April, there is worldwide recognition of autism. Because of the efforts of Autism Speaks, April is International Autism Awareness Month, as designated by the United Nations General Assembly in 2007. That was the same year that the US Congress recognized April as the month for autism awareness and called for more research into the causes of autism.[1]

Like something on a par with V-E Day in 1945, on Autism Speaks' website, people can read, "Every year, autism organizations around the world celebrate the day with unique fundraising and awareness-raising events."

Autism Speaks asks, "How will you celebrate?"

In 2012, I received an email from Autism Speaks that said, "Join Autism Speaks as we celebrate on April 2. Whether it's your front porch or city hall, an office party or a banquet, the whole world is going blue to increase awareness about autism.

"Last year, more than 70,000 people pledged to Light It Up Blue to shine a light on autism for World Autism Awareness Day."

One line on their site showed scenes of famous places all around the world flooded with blue lights to add to the festivities. Among the landmarks were the Paris Stock Exchange, Al Anoud Tower, Riyadh, Saudi Arabia, the New York Stock Exchange, Rockefeller Center and the Empire State Building in New York City, the statute of Christ the Redeemer in Brazil, the Great Buddha at Hyogo in Japan, the Sydney Opera House in Australia, and even Niagara Falls.

The email featured the photo of a smiling mother with an adorable little girl who was also smiling. There wasn't much explanation given on what exactly we have to celebrate, and, after reading countless autism stories in the news, I think a more appropriate color for the month would be black.

On Autism Awareness Day in 2013, the Secretary-General of the UN, Ban Ki-moon, delivered his annual message on autism. (He is from South Korea and became the Secretary General of the UN in 2007.)[2]

His message has been largely unchanged since 2008: All we need is attention, inclusion, awareness, support, understanding, and commitment. I wonder if Ban Ki-moon noticed that when he became Secretary-General in 2007, the autism rate was one in every 150 children, and today it's one in 50 children. There wasn't any alarm over the ever-increasing numbers. There was no call for answers. No acknowledgement of how severely many children are impacted by autism or any mention of the cost. It seems his message is scripted according to CDC guidelines: sound concerned, but never call autism a crisis.

The same is true of the press in the US, especially in April, when we're all supposed to be talking about awareness. Last year, in April 2013, there were a number of stories about autism published around the US. They typically called for awareness.

The numbers they reported were jaw-dropping, but no one demanded answers. Autism is best represented by the colorful puzzle-piece logo we're all so used to seeing.

On April 20, 2013, the paper *Morning Call,* in Lehigh Valley, Pennsylvania, published an article: "Walk Unites Families Touched by Autism."[3]

"More than 10,000 people flooded Dorney Park in South Whitehall Township on Saturday for Walk Now for Autism Speaks, the Lehigh Valley's largest such event."

Readers were told that participants, many with personal experience dealing with autism, came from throughout the area. Parents of two autistic sons were cited in the article. They described the diagnoses the boys have, including autism, sensory-processing disorder and oppositional defiant disorder. The parents were described as "overwhelmed" by the disability.

One sentence was especially concerning: "At age 3, Talon, a once-talkative child, abruptly stopped talking, reverting to biting and grunting." The other son didn't regress, but by the time he was 3, "rage took over."

The piece was typical of the coverage for Autism Awareness Month. The reporter acknowledged that the numbers were growing and that there was a need for awareness and support.

We're now used to hearing that there's been an increase and that kids can develop normally and suddenly become autistic. It's just part of the mystery of autism. Nowhere in this piece was the cause of autism talked about. The message was clear: autism happens, we don't know why, we need awareness.

Many parents believe that April should be Autism Action Month. Awareness is not enough. Celebrating seems callous in light of the very real problems facing people dealing with autism and the failure of the medical community and health officials to tell us anything conclusive about autism, other than the fact that vaccines don't cause it.

April coverage is designed to make us feel good about autism. There are lots of stories about local community events and nothing to make us worry about why so many children have an autism label today.

The disorder with no known cause, prevention, or cure, whose rate keeps inexplicably increasing, is never bad enough to cause real concern. On the Centers for Disease Control and Prevention website, they seem very knowledgeable about autism.[4] They also admit that a perfectly normal child can suddenly lose learned skills for no obvious reason and end up with autism.

"ASDs begin before the age of three and last throughout a person's life, although symptoms may improve over time. Some children with an ASD show hints of future problems within the first few months of life. In others, symptoms might not show up until twenty-four months or later. Some children with an ASD seem to develop normally until around eighteen to twenty-four months of age, and then they stop gaining new skills, or they lose the skills they once had."

They "seem to develop normally until around eighteen to twenty-four months of age and . . . lose the skills they once had" should be a warning given to every mother. Just because your baby can talk, make eye contact, and even be potty trained is not a guarantee. They could end up as a non-verbal autistic teenager in diapers. It's all just part of the puzzle of autism.

The CDC website has a question-and-answer section on autism and one of the questions is: "Is there an ASD epidemic?"[4]

The CDC's answer: "More people than ever before are being diagnosed with an ASD. It is unclear exactly how much of this increase is due to a broader definition of ASDs and better efforts in diagnosis. However, a true increase in the number of people with an ASD cannot be ruled out. We believe the increase in the diagnosis of ASDs is likely due to a combination of these factors.

"CDC is working with partners to study the prevalence of ASDs over time, so that we can find out if the number of children with these disorders is rising, dropping, or staying the same.

"We do know that ASDs are more common than we thought before and should be considered an important public health concern."

That's not really an answer, of course. It's an admission that the top health officials in the US don't know why a child regresses or why another child never develops speech. It may always have been like this. Doctors may have just misdiagnosed these children as something else in the past. It may be because the definition of autism is broader. Regardless, the CDC is interested in autism.

"ASDs continue to be an important public health concern. Like the many families living with ASDs, CDC wants to find out what causes the disorder. Understanding the risk factors that make a person more likely to develop an ASD will help us learn more about the causes."

And most of the official research involves genetics and poor choices/bad behavior on the part of the parents—especially the mother. That includes moms who drink, smoke, have babies too close together, have induced labor, marry older dads, have bad antibodies, are overweight, or who live too close to freeways.

It doesn't seem to bother officials at the CDC that after twenty years of having no answers, they still don't know anything.

"We do not know all of the causes of ASDs. However, we have learned that there are likely many causes for multiple types of ASDs. There may be many different factors that make a child more likely to have an ASD, including environmental, biologic, and genetic factors."

So it's all just a complicated mystery. Meanwhile there's so much autism everywhere that it's impossible to ignore it.

Pity the parents who rely on the official websites of CDC or AAP for answers.

There is never a consensus about autism. Top medical experts and government health officials will sometimes tell us that yes, the numbers are increasing. Sometimes, they're not. The claim that all the autism is the result of the broader definition they came up with in 1994 and not a real increase is alive and well.

In a *Huffington Post* piece on June 30, 2009, by Dr. Harvey Karp, the message was much different.[5] Karp was described as "a world-renowned child-development expert and America's most read pediatrician" in "Cracking the Autism Riddle: Toxic Chemicals, A Serious Suspect in the Autism Outbreak." He wrote: "Within three to four years, we expect to have enough data accumulated to start detecting what chemicals might be linked to autism." The National Children's Study (NCS) would be looking at the relationship between chemicals and other health problems like diabetes, cancer, birth defects, and infertility, which also are increasing, according to Karp.

Then Karp called for some very specific and controversial research:

"Beside the NCS, I support other new studies to look at: 1) the autism risk in vaccinated vs. unvaccinated kids; 2) the metabolism of vaccine ingredients (like aluminum, added to make shots work better), 3) more accurate determinations of the true incidence of autism. (The number of kids getting autism is unclear. Some studies suggest that much of the autism spike is just a 'labeling shift': kids who used to be labeled 'mentally retarded' increasingly are being labeled as 'autistic.')."

Karp's comments must have sent shockwaves through mainstream medicine. He was a regular speaker at AAP events around the US. If "America's most-read pediatrician" was talking about toxins and autism, then those calling it a solely genetic disorder were wrong. Lots of people in high places had gone on the record holding fast to the claim that we've always had so many autistic kids everywhere; we just didn't call it autism.

If this prominent doctor wanted to see a vaccinated vs. unvaccinated study done, along with studies on vaccine ingredients, maybe there was something to the vaccine-autism claim.

Karp's remarks came at a time when America was in the grip of an ever-increasing autism rate.

One in 150 US Children has Autism.

When the CDC finally got around to releasing the update on the autism rate from one in 166 to one in every 150 children/one in every 94 boys in February 2007 (based on outdated study numbers from 2000 and 2002), they did so still denying any real increase.

Dr. Marshalyn Yeargin-Allsopp, chief of the CDC's developmental-disabilities program at the National Center on Birth Defects and Developmental Disabilities, said at the time that the increase in the rate from one in 166 to one in 150 didn't really mean "the rates of autism have gone up, just that now we have some more definitive data."[6]

Former head of the CDC, Dr. Julie Gerberding, agreed that autism isn't more common, it's just that "our estimates are becoming better and more consistent, though we can't yet tell if there is a true increase in ASDs or if the changes are the result of our better studies."[7]

Dr. Paul Offit, America's most often cited expert on the autism-vaccine controversy, explained that the increase in autism is due to the fact that "people that we once called quirky or geeky or nerdy are now called autistic."[8]

In the *New York Times* article "Study Puts Rate of Autism at 1 in 150 US Children," by Benedict Carey, Dr. Fred R. Volkmar, from Yale University School of Medicine, was quoted as saying, "It appears that the rates are unchanged over the past twenty years or so."[8]

Lots of top experts seemed solidly behind the "no real increase" mantra. Yet, Karp said all the kids with autism meant there were environmental triggers. This was a major happening. Karp pointed to endocrine-disrupting chemicals (EDCs) as the culprits causing so many kids to be autistic. Karp wrote on *Huffington,* "In recent years, research has mounted against a virtual police lineup of EDCs, like BPA (in food cans, hard plastic water bottles), phthalates (in soft plastics, cosmetics) and fire retardants (in sofas, computers, flame-resistant clothing)."

Those who admit that toxins in the environment could possibly be at fault don't include the poisons regularly injected into babies and small children in their mandated vaccination schedule. Teflon, plastics, and formaldehyde should be worrying everyone, not the mercury, formaldehyde, and aluminum in vaccines.

## One in 110 US Children Has Autism

On Dec. 18, 2009, when the rate reached one in 110, NBC News quoted Catherine Rice, one of the researchers in the study, who was still unsure what the number meant. "At this point, it's impossible to say how much is a true increase and how much is identification."[9]

Rice made it clear that the cause was unknown but offered assurance that doctors were working on genetics and environmental triggers. While not sounding alarmed, she also didn't offer much hope that answers would be forthcoming. "Results from the environmental research are still years away," Rice said.

The NBC News video announced that the CDC believes autism is considered "a significant public health concern."

Dr. Max Wiznitzer, from the Rainbow Babies & Children's Hospital of Cleveland, was shown making it clear that "this study does not tell us the 'why.' It just tells us what's going on, and it identifies a public health issue."

The next segment of the report had Wiznitzer telling parents about the warning signs they should look for, like loss of speech and eye contact.

This must have made a lot of viewers uneasy. It's one thing to have a child who never develops language and other skills, but what Wiznitzer meant was that a child who can speak can inexplicably stop talking. NBC was warning parents that no child, even a healthy one, is safe from autism.

## One in 88 US Children Has Autism

Three years later, on March 29, 2012, CDC Director Thomas Frieden announced a new autism rate of one in every 88 children. This was not done at a well-publicized press conference but during a hastily announced conference call. Rather than face the cameras and advise the nation that we're in the grip of yet another dramatic increase in autism, he chose this low-key way to give us the news. The message remained the same: We can't say how much might be a real increase. Agency spokespeople were out in force, assuring everyone that officials were looking into the situation.

That same day, CNN quoted Frieden: "How much of that increase is a result of better tracking and how much of it is a result of an actual increase, we still don't know. We know more about autism today than we have ever known, but there is still so much we don't know and wish that we knew."[10]

The CDC's Dr. Coleen Boyle talked about "accelerating our research into risk factors and causes of autism-spectrum disorders."[11] Despite the fact that the autism rate had doubled in six years, Dr. Boyle didn't seem worried during the interview. She merely said, "No matter what the number is, there's one thing for certain, and that is more children are being identified with autism."

*LA Times*: "Autism researchers around the country said the CDC data—including striking geographic and racial variations in the rates and how they have changed—suggest that rising awareness of the disorder, better detection, and improved access to services can explain much of the surge, and perhaps all of it."[12]

*Reuters*: "There is a good possibility that much of the reported increase in the prevalence of autism is illusory, however. When asked about this during the news conference, CDC's Frieden pointed out that 'doctors have gotten better at diagnosing the condition, and communities have gotten better at providing services, so I think we can say it is possible that the increase is the result of better detection.'"[13]

ABC News: "But what this rise actually means is still a mystery. Some doctors contacted by ABC News believe a broader definition of autism has contributed to rising rates."[14]

Dr. Isabelle Rapin, professor of pediatrics and neurology at the Albert Einstein College of Medicine, was cited by ABC. She stated that the diagnostic criteria had changed, which was why more children are labeled autistic today than they were ten or twenty years ago. According to Rapin, doctors, parents, teachers, and the public in general are all better at recognizing autism.

The press gave the new autism number lots of coverage, yet no one seemed willing to ask uncomfortable questions like:

When will officials be able to explain what's happening?

How could this still be due to a broader criteria for autism, when the definition was expanded back in 1994?

Why is the autism rate always based on studies of children?

Where are the autistic adults?

How could this be a genetic disorder if the rate is continually increasing?

Regardless, the official explanation was the same as usual.

March 29, 2012, a *Washington Post* article by David Brown announced, "The rising rate of autism could be the result of finding children missed in earlier surveys or an actual increase in the condition—or a combination of the two. The trend has been observed in Canada and Western Europe as well as the United States."[15]

"In a telephone briefing with reporters, Thomas Frieden, CDC's director, said the increase could be 'the result of better detection." Brown quoted Frieden, who called for early detection and treatment.

*The Washington Post* did include Mark Roithmayr, president of Autism Speaks at that time, who strongly disagreed with Frieden. Roithmayr said that autism was "becoming an epidemic," and he called for "a national plan." He dissented from those who said it was merely better diagnosing.

On the same day, a *New York Times* story by Benedict Carey on March 29, 2012, did everything to convince readers that nothing was really new here.[16]

"The frequency of autism-spectrum diagnoses has been increasing for decades, but researchers cannot agree on whether the trend is a result of heightened awareness, an expanding definition of the spectrum, an actual increase in incidence, or some combination of those factors." Carey said that diagnosing autism "is not an exact science" and that the spectrum takes in a wide variety of affected children. He pointed out that there were experts who feel that children who get "extensive state-financed support services" might be a factor in the new rate.

Carey continued to downplay the impact autism was having by noting that a new definition of autism in 2013 would possibly reduce the rate. In addition, he quoted Dr. Éric Fombonne, a psychiatrist at McGill University in Montreal, who said that this study couldn't really show if there was a true increase.

As if to drive home the point, the *New York Times* had another story on the new rate a week later, April 7, 2012. This one was by Amy Harmon, and the title was "The Autism Wars." In the first paragraph she announced, "The CDC said it was possible that the increase could be entirely attributed to better detection by teachers and doctors, while holding out the possibility of unknown environmental factors."[17]

Harmon speculated on a number of things that could be responsible for the autism increase. It may be just part of a popular trend, and she quoted a commenter on the first *Times* story. "Just like how all of a sudden everyone had ADHD in the nineties, now everyone has autism." Perhaps the definition was just too broad.

The rest of the piece talked about how variable the diagnosis is and speculated on the number of adults with autism.

On March 29, 2012 Diane Sawyer at ABC News called the announcement "a staggering medical headline today about autism."[18] The one in 88 figure represented a twenty-five percent increase, and she sounded very concerned.

Sawyer talked to ABC's medical advisor, Dr. Richard Besser, who called it "a startling increase." Besser showed viewers a video of a little girl and described her as "a perfectly healthy child until she was fifteen months old." Her mother then said, "When I called her name, she didn't turn around anymore." Besser said only, "Classic signs, autism. Nobody knows what causes it."

Next, Dr. Besser talked with Dr. Gary Goldstein. Again, there was no alarm over the numbers. Besser asked Goldstein what it was like twenty years ago compared to today. Goldstein said that they had "about a hundred patients with autism coming in for evaluation," and now they have 2,000.

When Besser asked him if more children have autism now or if the increase is due to better diagnosing, Goldstein said that the answer to both questions is "Yes." Nothing more was said about the increase. Instead, Besser simply added that "No one knows why." He also said that boys have an autism rate five times greater than girls do, again with no explanation.

Besser's upbeat coverage continued. He said the "good news" is that there's more early intervention and that kids are making improvement. As this was said, viewers were shown happy children interacting with therapists. Meanwhile, nothing was said about why a child stops talking and making eye contact in the first place.

Back in the studio, Diane Sawyer didn't seem as casual about the new numbers as Dr. Besser. She said, "Rich, we just heard the terrifying phrase, not only more diagnoses, but more autism. Why? What is going on?"

Besser quickly jumped in, citing better detection, and then he called for more research. "Until we know what causes autism, it's very hard to say why we're seeing really more cases."

What ABC presented to parents during this autism-rate update was a very chilling example of regressive autism. Your child might be born healthy and appear to have normal development, but suddenly they can stop responding and end up with autism. That can result in years of intense behavioral therapy that could cost your family their life's savings. That's simply the way it is with autism. There's nothing we can do to prevent it.

In a March 29 report from NBC by AP reporter Mike Stobbe headline was "Better diagnosis, screening behind rise in autism."[19] Autism may be twice as common as it was just five years ago, but NBC was quick to say, "Health officials attribute the increase largely to better recognition of cases, through wide screening and better diagnosis."

Parents were cautioned that that are no easy answers when it comes to autism and that "the search for the cause of autism is really only beginning."

Stobbe included other experts with differing viewpoints. Dr. Coleen Boyle from the CDC admitted they didn't know why the numbers increased. Dr. Geraldine Dawson from Autism Speaks was adamant that things were bad. She said autism was now "a public health emergency that demands immediate attention."

At the end of the piece, Stobbe brought up the vaccine controversy. He quoted Dr. Arthur Caplan, director of the University of Pennsylvania's Center for Bioethics, who said we need to find out why the numbers continue to increase but that this continued increase was proof of no link to vaccines. "The rate of growth is simply inconsistent with anything having to do with vaccination."

So, if it's not vaccines, what is it? Caplan didn't speculate on what it might be.

Stobbe ended his article telling readers about the role of genetics in autism and research involving a possible link to the medications women take while pregnant. He said findings would be published in 2013.

## One in 50 US Children Has Autism

As if things weren't confusing enough, in March 2013, officials released another jaw-dropping number. Mike Stobbe reported that according to one study, the real rate was one in fifty US children.[20] The usual caveat was included, "Health officials say the new number doesn't mean autism is occurring more often. But it does suggest that doctors are diagnosing autism more frequently, especially in children with milder problems."

On March 20, *US News* released the story "One in 50 School-Aged Children in US Has Autism: CDC—Significant increase in the prevalence of the condition over the past five years, researchers say" by Steven Reinberg.[21]

Reinberg quoted Stephen Blumberg, a senior scientist at the CDC, who wasn't too concerned. "This estimate was a bit surprising. There may be more children with autism-spectrum disorder than previously thought." In order to give people an accurate image of what this meant, Blumberg suggested that if the average school bus holds fifty students, "typically one child with autism-spectrum disorder is on every full school bus in America." All this was due to "better diagnosing."

Blumberg stated "improved ascertainment" was behind the shocking new figure.

Autism Speaks' Michael Rosanoff was cited saying that this was proof that previous figures had "underestimated the real prevalence of autism."

Reinberg, the author of the piece, said nothing about any action officials were planning to take in the face of yet another stunning new autism statistic.

*New York Daily News*, March 29, 2013.[22] In a piece called "One in Fifty American kids has autism: What the latest figures tell us," was a photo of six-year-old twins, Ariana and Feriyal Khan, smiling and hugging during a ballet class. The story said, "Although National Autism Awareness Month doesn't officially start until Monday, the campaign got a jump-start last week with the finding that autism-spectrum disorders, or ASDs, affect 1 in 50 American children, according to the Centers for Disease Control and Prevention." The story continued telling readers this was "a significant increase" from the last update of one in every 88, but it was difficult to compare the two rates because there were "different methods" of research involved. According to the CDC, "Both reports help paint a more complete picture of autism in our nation."

*The Daily News* also expressed concern. "In either case, the data shows skyrocketing reports of these disorders among children, with boys four times as likely as girls to be diagnosed. The extent to which these rates reflect a better understanding and, thus, diagnosing of these conditions is unknown, but 'a true increase in the number of people with an ASD cannot be ruled out,' the CDC says on its website."

Michael Rosanoff, epidemiologist and associate director for public health research at Autism Speaks, was cited in the story. He felt that we've been "underestimating the magnitude of this public health challenge." At least half the increase was something besides better diagnosing, according to Rosanoff.

Again, no one could explain why the numbers continued to go up; at the same time, no one seemed worried about the possibility of a real increase in a disorder without a known cause, prevention, or cure.

Other important news outlets covered it.

CBS News had a twenty-one second report on March 20, 2013, where the news anchor concluded, "The new numbers may simply be the result of better reporting."[23]

That same day, *NBC Nightly News* anchor Brian Williams merely said, "The number of children with autism in this country may be a lot higher than previously thought, according to new research from the CDC."[24]

NBC medical expert Dr. Robert Bazell continued the story: "Autism diagnoses have grown to the point where parents report fully one in fifty school-aged children has autism."

A mom was shown saying that this was scary and that someone should figure out why this is happening.

Bazell pointed out that one in fifty children with a diagnosis of autism didn't mean that there'd been "a genuine increase in the neurological changes that are labeled as autism." He added that the new numbers meant that there were now a million autistic children in the US.

Next, Dr. Zachary Warren, from Vanderbilt University Medical Center, appeared, telling viewers about factors like changing awareness and better recognition that could explain the new rate.

As happy children were shown climbing on playground equipment, a voiceover from Bazell said, "Experts say more research is needed to know for certain whether other factors are involved in the ever-growing numbers of American children being diagnosed with autism."

The largest advocacy group, Autism Speaks, neatly explained the supposed increase.[25] "A new government survey of parents indicates that one in fifty school-aged children have autism-spectrum disorder (ASD). This is significantly higher than the official government estimate of one in eighty-eight American children. It also supports research suggesting that many affected children are being missed by the surveillance methods the Centers for Disease Control (CDC) uses to produce its official estimate.

"As far as the competing rate of one in every 88 children, Michael Rosanoff said, 'This number does not replace the official one in eighty-eight estimate, but it does suggest that it may be a significant underestimate of autism prevalence in the US.'"

*Forbes*: "Children [who] were, therefore, walking around for quite a few years with autism that went unrecognized and uncounted. That fits with the idea that a lot of the increase in autism we've seen in the last decade has much to do with greater awareness and identification."[26]

*New York Times*: "According to experts not involved in the report, the increase coincided with a period of soaring awareness of autism-spectrum disorders among clinicians and schools, as well as parents.[27]

'The report emphasized that while the numbers changed from 1 in 88 children, ages 6 to 17, having received a diagnosis in a 2007 parent survey, to 1 in 50 children in the current report, most of the increase was because of previously undiagnosed cases."

*Reuters*: "As many as one in 50 US school-aged children have a diagnosis of autism, up 72 percent since 2007, but much of the increase involves milder cases, suggesting the rise is linked to better recognition of autism symptoms and not more cases, government researchers said on Wednesday."[28]

The overall message was that nothing was wrong with having an autism rate of two percent of children. There was a good explanation: More kids didn't really have autism. In 2012, one in eighty-eight was no real increase, either.

What's really hard to figure out is the fact that when the rate went from 1 in 110 to 1 in 88 back in March 2012, everyone was saying the same thing about the increase. All the major news sources denied a true increase. In fact, that was the standard explanation whenever the rate was updated.

The numbers continued to worsen, and, again, officials showed no surprise or alarm. On March 27, 2014, the CDC announced a new national autism rate of one in every sixty-eight children. It was quickly covered by all the major news outlets *USA Today*:

> "Autism rates climbed nearly 30 percent between 2008 and 2010 and have more than doubled since the turn of the century, according to a new study from the US Centers for Disease Control and Prevention."[29] The report said that a rate of one in every 68 children meant that "virtually every grade in every elementary school has at least one child with autism—a seemingly astonishing rise for a condition that was nearly unheard of a generation ago." *USA Today* may have called it "a seemingly astonishing rise," but they were quick to tell readers that a lot of experts felt it was "better awareness and diagnosis," and not really more kids with autism. The CDC's Coleen Boyle again had no answers. "Our system tells us what's going on. It (only) gives us clues as to the 'why.'"
>
> As if to assure the public this wasn't something to worry about, *USA Today* cited the fact that "experts said they were not surprised by the increase."

There were findings that said the rate would "continue to climb," according to Dr. Walter Zahorodny, a psychologist from Rutgers who directed the New Jersey Autism Study. "To me, it seems like autism prevalence can only get higher," he said.

CDC officials like Coleen Boyle were quoted in numerous stories.

CNN:

"'The report is not designed to say why more children are being diagnosed with autism,'" Boyle says. But she believes increased awareness in identifying and diagnosing children contributes to the higher numbers."[30]

Notice Dr. Boyle said that "the number of children diagnosed with autism continues to rise," not the number of children with autism. She still claimed it was all just being aware of a condition that's always been around.

NBC News:

> The latest look at autism in the US shows a startling 30 percent jump among eight-year-olds diagnosed with the disorder in a two-year period, to one in every sixty-eight children.[31]
>
> The Centers for Disease Control and Prevention, which did the survey, says the numbers almost certainly reflect more awareness and diagnosis of kids who would have been missed in years past.

Coleen Boyle again made the claim that the number of children with a diagnosis had increased—not the incidence of autism.

NBC cited Max Wiznitzer, who said that one in 68 was "a rise in diagnosis," not in autism.

Other experts joined in support of the claim of no real increase. Dr. Lisa Shulman, a specialist in autism at the Albert Einstein College of Medicine at Yeshiva University in New York, said that it was better identification.

NBC neatly made the case that if a top official and leading experts don't see anything new happening, everything was under control.

Interestingly, Dr. Alvarez at Fox didn't agree with the claim of no real increase. While he didn't go so far as to use the word "crisis" to describe the situation, he did said the rate update was "shocking."

Fox News:

> Even if you take into consideration the more aggressive screenings, where in some cases, there might have been a misdiagnosis, I still feel that this continues to be a wake-up

> call for parents, teachers, pediatricians, and the federal government to better identify children on the spectrum, since the only effective tool for treatment we have is early intervention. Also, the discrepancy from state to state might give more weight to environmental factors as a cause.[32]

And in an amazing story from *Philly.com*, Walter Zahorodny talked about what the new rate meant. Zahorodny, who was in charge of the numbers collected in New Jersey, said 'The new report should put to rest the argument over whether the increase in autism diagnoses stems from growing awareness or reflects growing numbers of children with the disabling condition.[33]

"It's a true increase,' he said. "It's a change of great magnitude. It's silly to go on debating that." Zahorodny restated the fact that he expected the numbers to get worse.

For a top researcher to emphatically say the increase was real was almost unheard of, and it was especially significant because back on April 2, 2012, on the *Brian Lehrer Show* on WNYC radio, Zahorodny acknowledged that for some kids, it was their vaccines: "Vaccines don't play a significant role in autism increasing. Some small number of children probably do have autism because of an adverse vaccine reaction, but they don't make for the overall rise."[34]

Despite being very cautious in his public comment, Zahorodny made it clear: there is a link.

This new rate announcement came out just before the beginning of April, Autism Awareness Month. Coincidentally, another study was announced at the same time.

On March 27, 2014, ABC 7 in Detroit ran the story, "STUDY: Autism likely caused by abnormal brain growth during pregnancy, not vaccines."[35]

In the news clip, a reporter said that a new post-mortem study of the brains of eleven children with autism revealed that signs of autism could be detected by the second trimester of a woman's pregnancy. Reporter: "If these results can hold in larger studies, researchers say the findings provide even stronger evidence that autism is caused by something before the child is born, not by something that happens to them later in life, like getting a vaccine."

This study, involving only eleven children, was reported on by most major news sources. Lead researcher Dr. Eric Courchesne, at the University of California, San Diego, had been researching prenatal signs of autism for years as his previous research had shown. By now, the public was used to convenient studies announced at the same time as an update in the autism rate—studies that pointed to something else besides vaccines.

Parents should have by now accepted the fact that no matter what the increase, no one in a position of authority would be able to explain why the numbers keep increasing, no numbers would ever be definitive, and no one would ever be worried.

Back on Oct. 6. 2013, there was a story by reporter Mark Roth of the *Pittsburgh Post Gazette* entitled "Debate continues: Is autism really growing?"[36]

It summed up the confusion over the numbers. Roth began the piece citing the rates of one in 88, one in 100, and one in 38. He told readers that these numbers "show the rate of autism in today's world." The huge differences between the statistics are clearly baffling. One in 88 is from the CDC, one in 100 is from a British study of autistic adults in 2011, and one in 38 comes from children in Korea, also in 2011.

The numbers make no sense. What's really going on? Why can't the agencies that receive millions of dollars a year to address our health tell us what's happening?

Mark Roth said, "The sharply different estimates add more fuel to the debate over how common autism is and whether it is on the rise. To show what a difference the varying estimates would make in Allegheny County alone, which has 1.2 million residents, the number of autistic people could range from 12,000, using the British figure, to more than 32,000, using the South Korea study."

It is no wonder, then, that leading autism researchers have conflicting opinions on how widespread the disorder is. Still—it isn't universally accepted that the numbers represent a true increase.

Roth wrote, "Among the scientists who believe autism is showing a real increase in America are Thomas Insel, the director of the National Institute of Mental Health; David Amaral, research director at the MIND Institute at the University of California at Davis; and Peter Bearman, a social sciences professor at Columbia University."

Dr. Insel, who's also the head of the Interagency Autism Coordinating Committee, created by Congress to deal with autism, discounted the idea that all the autism is just better diagnosing of a disorder that's always been around. In a stunning statement, Insel said, "There is a large proportion of people with this disorder who are so disabled that it is unthinkable to me that they weren't detected in the past. If you have a twelve-year-old in diapers who is head banging and has no language, it's hard for me to believe these kids existed in 1980 and were not being labeled."

Roth presented both sides of the argument, citing Terry Brugha, of the University of Leicester in England, who believes that the autism rate has always been around one percent of the population, and his adult survey confirmed this.

Dr. David Amaral of the MIND Institute at the University of California-Davis disagreed and said he felt that the increase was real. There were environmental causes, and he urged people "to stay open to whatever influences there might be and be willing to explore them."

This article could only add to the confusion. It was clear that there was nothing about autism that experts could agree on.

Roth cited Dr. Nancy Minshew, the University of Pittsburgh didn't see any problem with all the autism everywhere and said she believes that in the past all the severe cases were placed in institutions. According to her, the increase was due to better recognition. In the past, we didn't include high-functioning people in the diagnosis.

Turning to the 2011 South Korean study, Roth admitted that the one in 38 South Korean rate might be alarming. The advocacy group Autism Speaks, which helped fund the South Korean study, speculated that maybe the US had underestimated the autism numbers. Maybe the rate was similar here. Roth noted that pediatrics professor Isaac Kohane of Harvard Medical School questioned the accuracy of the Korean study.

Roth said that there should be a study done across the population to get the true rate for autism but that the CDC wasn't interested in doing this type of broad-based study on autism, "for whatever reason," according to Thomas Insel. Roth left readers with the ominous prediction that "the debate on the true numbers of autistic people in the United States will likely continue for years."

Despite the numbers, federal health officials clearly didn't intend to make autism a priority. The statistics would remain part of the puzzle we call autism. Members of the press knew this. No one was going to hold officials accountable, especially those speaking out in the media. They'd be allowed to continue guessing about autism.

Why didn't Mark Roth pursue the issue further? How many more years would officials be allowed to claim that autism has always been here like this? Why don't reporters demand to know why no one is able to show us the forty-, fifty-, and sixty-year-olds who displayed the same signs of classic autism we see in so many of our children? Why do members of the media refuse to hold these people accountable for what's happening to our children?

It was interesting that Thomas Insel was convinced that the autism rate was really increasing by Oct. 2013. He'd given conflicting messages in the past.

On August 5, 2009, the Senate Appropriations Subcommittee, chaired by Senator Tom Harkin, held a hearing on the state of autism research, treatments and interventions in the US.[37]

A number of autism experts and parents addressed the senators. Two speakers exemplified the controversy that rages in this country over vaccines and autism. One was Thomas Insel, M.D., director of the National Institute of Mental Health and chairman of the Interagency Autism Coordinating Committee (IACC); the other was Dana Halverson, co-founder of BEAT-Iowa and mother of Robin, her seven-year-old daughter with autism.

Sen. Harkin opened the hearing talking about autism. He made it clear: Autism has environmental triggers, and "the rate of incidence is growing." He also said we have to look at "how to address the needs of the growing population of adults with autism."

Insel testified first. He gave an overview of autism with the standard definitions we've all heard over and over. He said 10 to 20 percent of autistic kids regress. "[They] seem to develop quite well for the first eighteen months and will clearly lose language, lose function."

Insel spent a lot of time talking about research on "genomics," "syndromes," and "rare but significant mutations," assuring us that there's "clearly a genetic factor at work here." He also feels that "we still need to learn how genes and environment interact."

Insel then turned his attention to the prevalence of autism. "The Centers for Disease Control and Prevention now reports from 2007 a rate of about one in every 150 children, eight-year-olds being given a diagnosis. That's about a tenfold increase over the numbers coming from the CDC from the 1992-1993 period."

He quickly added, "The tenfold increase in prevalence is of great interest to many of us. I just want to just caution you that a change in prevalence is not unique to autism. We've seen a fortyfold increase in the prevalence of pediatric bipolar disorder over the same period. We've seen perhaps a tenfold or greater increase in attention deficit hyperactivity disorder in children over the last three or four decades."

Insel's lack of concern over these increases was evident. He gave no reason for the changes except to say, "We have to remember the difference between prevalence, which can be affected by ascertainment, by changes in diagnosis, and the difference in incidence, which we don't have right now, good evidence that there's a true increase in the incidence ... the rate of new cases." He added, "That's an area that requires more research."

Despite the explosive rate, Insel was trying to convince the committee that he was still not sure if autism has really increased. In the face of parents testifying over a lack of services and bankrupting costs, Insel tried to pretend that all this autism is nothing new. How many more years are officials going to scratch their heads over the autism rate? The CDC gets billions to run health care in the US, and they can't give us the current rate of autism. It was slightly disingenuous of Insel to say that the rate of one in 150 was from eight-year-olds in 2007. Certainly someone in his position knows that rate is from studies done in 2000 and 2002 but not released until 2007.

Back in 2007, when the CDC announced their updated autism figures, I wrote "The Really Big Lie About Autism" to show that no matter how bad the numbers, officials will never admit that there are really more kids with autism. Insel's comments are proof that the lie has remained alive and well.

In December 2009, Insel spoke at MIT.[38] This was four months after he testified on autism before US Senator Tom Harkin's subcommittee. In August, Insel still wasn't sure if there are really more kids with autism, but by December, he was convinced—the increase is real.

One percent of children officially had autism in 2009. Insel acknowledged that something in the environment is responsible for this global explosion in a neuro-developmental disorder, and he readily admitted he has no clue what is behind it. Insel's MIT speech epitomized this paralysis.

Whenever Insel talks about autism, he has a smiling, relaxed manner. He's in charge of a federal committee created by Congress to address autism, and he's spent years telling us he knows nothing.

At MIT, Insel presented his usual autism powerpoint slides and went through the standard autism info. He defined autism. He showed videos of a normally progressing baby who regressed into autism between one year and eighteen months and ended up as a non-verbal fourteen-year-old. This regression was described by Insel as "really a very interesting problem which we don't fully understand."

Insel presented slides of brain scans and DNA strands and talked about genetics. He said that 10 percent of cases have a genetic link. Besides bad genes, paternal age was also a factor.

In talking about the genetics of autism, Insel used words like "spectacular," "striking," and "amazing."

In the end, he had to admit that genes "won't explain all cases."

Next Insel turned to prevalence. He said the debate over the numbers is a "very interesting discussion." He reminisced about the difficulty of finding a child with autism thirty years ago. "I'd never seen any children with autism through all of my training. . . . I didn't actually know anyone that I trained with who'd actually seen a child with autism."

He said he'd seen the data from *Pediatrics*, the official journal of the American Academy of Pediatrics, putting the current rate at one in ninety, but he admitted that he didn't know how to interpret that rate. Insel was also unsure about what was driving this, but he was sure it wasn't diagnostic substitution.

It sounded like he was talking about a real crisis. A shocking number of our children now have a disorder that was previously unknown. Insel couldn't tell us why, and there's no way to prevent more children from becoming victims. Amazingly, Insel wasn't worried that the one in ninety rate might get worse.

"I said before this isn't just genetics. . . . There have to be environmental factors. . . . We have barely been able to scratch the surface. . . . There are something like 80,000 potential toxicants." Insel talked about prenatal exposures to toxins.

His Powerpoint presentation included slides with questions: "Environmental Influences in Autism: What do we need? . . . Why do we care?"

Insel never really addressed the "Why do we care?" question, but he ended the lecture talking about lots of things, from better detection and intervention to having more studies.

He kept showing brain scans of children and talking about neuro-imaging while saying he still didn't know very much. He did say he believes autism is really "Ten, twenty, forty disorders."

As far as what the environmental exposure behind autism might be, Insel was at a loss. The one thing he was sure of was that vaccines don't cause autism.

"The only thing I would argue has actually been investigated with any rigor, and even then it's limited, is the vaccine hypothesis. There have been these very extensive epidemiological studies of vaccines and autism, in France, in Denmark, in the United States, hundreds of thousands of children included. That's actually, surprisingly, come up empty-handed." He went on to describe research on thimerosal, which he described as a "neurotoxin" that was used in vaccines until 2001. There wasn't a subsequent drop in the autism rate, therefore, "you can certainly say it's not driving this huge increase."

So many things have changed since the 1980s, according to Insel. Smiling broadly, he told us that the list is enormous and that we've barely begun to crack the surface.

During the questions after his talk, a dad in the audience challenged Insel on the claim that the mercury was removed from *all* vaccines in 2001. Insel quickly admitted that the dad was right—it's still in the flu shot and maybe some others.

The dad brought up aluminum in vaccines. Insel didn't address it.

The dad asked why polio was an emergency for the US when it affected one in 5,000 people, but one percent of children with autism isn't. Insel ignored the question.

Instead, Insel tried to change the subject. Throwing up his arms, Insel lamented, "My argument is that there are about 900 things we could be looking at, and that is the only thing we've looked at so far, at least epidemiologically. The signal isn't there yet."

He said he didn't want "to get wrapped around that issue" and called for looking into other things.

Next the questioner brought up biomedical treatment and recovery. He said his autistic son recovered with biomedical help. The father wanted to know why Insel wasn't interested in this. He said the children with autism are "sick kids."

Insel jumped on the topic. "We've just launched a study of recovery. I couldn't agree with you more. This field came . . . I couldn't agree with you more." He sounded excited as he talked about blaming "refrigerator mothers" thirty years ago. According to Insel, autism was "a biological problem" that is connected to other systems in the body.

If it hadn't been for the audience, Insel wouldn't have brought up the study of biomedical treatment and recovery. He didn't mention it in the talk, only at the questions at the end.

Insel talked as if the whole controversy over vaccines was about thimerosal. He knows that's not the case, but it's easier to sell his message if he covers up how involved this issue really is.

Insel may be able to dismiss the vaccine link and dilute the topic by talking about genes and older dads, but those numbers continue to haunt him. Very soon, autism won't be just a health care issue. It's going to an economic crisis for this country. A massive, dependent population of young autistic adults is about to descend on the US. Insel knows this. He quietly admits it, but he does it at places like MIT and NIH. Insel isn't on ABC News telling us the increase is real.

Then in 2010, during an hour-and-a-half-long speech at the National Institute of Health, Dr. Insel discussed what scientists know about autism. He said that if one in ninety children has autism, it means that there are about 700,000 children in this country with autism.[39] Furthermore he added, "Eighty percent of the people with a diagnosis of autism in the US are under the age of eighteen." Insel described it as "a huge wave that is moving through the system."

This was alarming information and rare for any official to talk about autism in these terms. Insel was at a loss to tell the audience why this is happening. He did make it clear that the claim of better diagnosing and expanded spectrum could explain only a small portion of the increase. He talked at length about environmental toxins being the cause of the soaring rate of autism. He also admitted he's clueless as to what the exact triggers might be. "What's probably more striking here is what we don't know."

Insel said that he and others had actually made a list of possible toxic exposures that might be behind the autism increase, and he named fluoride and fertilizers as examples of what they came up with. In the end, they came to no conclusions.

What really got my attention was a passing comment he made about what the future holds for this country. In Insel's own words, "We have responded to this as if it's a crisis. We see this as an enormous public health challenge. If you look at those numbers, the increase, and recognize how many of those kids will become adults, we . . . also need to be thinking about how we prepare the nation for a million people who may need significant amounts of services as they are no longer cared for by their parents or as their parents are no longer around."

Insel did not actually call autism "a crisis." He said, "as if it's a crisis." No one at the Centers for Disease Control and Prevention or the American Academy of Pediatrics has ever referred to autism as "a crisis." "Public health challenge" is the strongest language ever used by officials at the CDC, and it looks like everyone in positions of authority has gotten the message that autism is merely a "challenge," never a "crisis."

To the average person, the idea of a million disabled adults overwhelming social services in the coming years seems more of a disaster/emergency than a crisis. In addition, Insel gave the audience no idea of how he intends to "prepare the nation" for the autism tsunami. Imagine what solutions he'll come up with to meet that challenge.

Insel added, "We need to figure out how this gets paid for and who provides the care." There was no alarm being sounded. He used the term "interesting" most often in referring to what they were finding out about autism. He's in the midst of this nightmare, charged with addressing what's happening to hundreds of thousands of children right before his eyes, yet he continues to scratch his head over what's behind the epidemic. Insel didn't hesitate to say over and over that "we don't know."

Insel began his talk by saying: "The best experts may be the parents," but he didn't say a word about the claim by countless thousands of parents that their children were healthy and normally developing until they received certain routine vaccinations.

Thomas Insel admitted this is an epidemic increase of disabled children. He pointed out that it's worldwide and that the numbers continue to grow. He's aware of what will happen to this nation when one percent of adults as well as children have autism. He readily acknowledged that he has no way of preventing more and more children from falling victim to autism. And he talked about all of this with no sense of real urgency.

On Monday, July 11, 2011, Dr. Thomas Insel, chairman of the Interagency Autism Coordinating Committee, testified before the US House of Representatives Energy and Commerce Subcommittee on Health in support of the reauthorization of the Combating Autism Act.[40]

Insel's 2011 testimony should be compared to what he said during the 2009 Senate hearing.

Back in August of 2009, Insel wasn't sure if the rate of autism was really going up or not. He talked about early diagnosis and early intervention. He talked about genetic research.

In December 2009, the autism rate officially went from one in every 150 children to one in every 110 kids. That same month, speaking at MIT, Insel said, "I said before this isn't just genetics . . . There have to be environmental factors."

By the spring of 2010, Insel was really getting concerned about the impact of autism. At the National Institutes of Health, he said, "Eighty percent of the people with a diagnosis of autism in the US are under the age of eighteen." In Insel's own words, "If you look at those numbers, the increase, and recognize how many of those kids will become adults, we . . . also need to be thinking about how we prepare the nation for a million people who may need significant amounts of services as they are no longer cared for by their parents or as their parents are no longer around."

When Insel appeared in Congress on July 11, 2011, he was expected to report on the advances that had been made since 2009. After his testimony, members of the Health Subcommittee may have wondered why it made sense to continue the work of the IACC.

Insel couldn't give any specific answers about the cause of autism. He talked at length about the genetics involved. He cited all the organizations and agencies focused on autism. He was quick to say that while environmental factors may be at work here, he had no idea what they might be. Regarding the possible triggers, he made a vague reference to things like fertilizers, antidepressants, and prenatal exposures.

Evidently, no one on the subcommittee had read Insel's previous testimony because they seemed quite willing to accept that when it comes to autism, no one knows anything.

Several questions were asked about how autism funds were being spent. And there were expressions of concern about the lifetime-care cost estimate of $3.2 million cited by Insel.

Insel described autism as "an urgent national health priority" in front of the subcommittee, and, yet, in the IACC's Strategic Plan for Autism Spectrum Disorder Research published in January 2009, autism was called "a national health emergency."

According to Insel's testimony, the rate is one in every 110 eight-year-olds today, which wasn't exactly correct, since that number comes from studies of eight-year-olds in 2006. He emphasized that we should talk about "autism spectrum disorders" rather than "autism." His demeanor was positive, and he smiled a lot. He struck a perfect balance; he sounded concerned about autism but not alarmed. He made it clear that advances are being made, but, at the same time, he couldn't specifically name one.

Insel tried to sound like everything was under control; we're getting close to finding answers. And surprisingly, congressional members at the hearing didn't demand answers. They listened to the same old recitation of the definition of autism that doesn't come close to describing what desperate situations thousands of families with autistic children across this country live with, and they willingly accepted that experts still don't know why any it's happening.

There was a lot missing in his testimony. There was no mention of the growing concern over a link between the ever-expanding vaccine schedule and autism. Not a word was said about the children who were healthy at birth and who suddenly and dramatically regressed following routine vaccinations. At the same time he ignored the vaccine controversy, Insel couldn't name any environmental factor that was definitely linked to autism.

Regarding the epidemic rate, Insel said they "were amazed at how frequently they're seeing autism." Insel never once used terms like "alarmed" or "crisis."

There were references to what autism is going to cost this country. Insel, referring to Michael Ganz's 2006 Harvard autism study, told members of the committee to multiply $3.2 million by 500,000, which was his estimate of the number of autistic people who will be in need of extensive services.[41]

Insel noted that there was a lack of services for adults, but he had no real information on how critical this need is. There was no mention of the waiting lists that are growing exponentially.

Finally, while Insel might go to MIT and NIH and say things like 80 percent of autistic Americans are under the age of eighteen and that "we need to prepare for a million people who may be in need of significant services," in Congress, he sounded more positive. He focused on all the effort being made to find answers for this baffling condition.

Everyone in the room seemed satisfied that, as one congressman said, Insel was giving them "state of the art" information about autism. I can only expect that on Insel's next trip to Capitol Hill, he'll be saying the same thing.

Insel: "Most people are hearing more about autism than they might ever have imagined. . . . Two decades ago . . .when I was in medical school, we probably didn't hear much about autism, but at this point, we are amazed by how frequently we're seeing autism in clinics, particularly in pediatric clinics, neuro-psychiatric clinics. The CDC's latest prevalence estimates are one in 110 children, that's one in seventy boys, that's amongst the eight-year-old cohort today being diagnosed with autism-spectrum disorder.

And it is therefore that the disorder has become an urgent national health priority."

Insel talked about how they encourage public participation, written comments, public comment at their meetings, and town hall meetings. He says there's a high level of transparency. "The IACC ensures a diversity of ideas and perspectives on ASD are brought to the table."

While they're required to meet only twice a year, Insel said that the IACC has been meeting about sixteen times annually.

Insel: "I think we've seen some remarkable progress in the identification of how common ASD is within communities, how ASD develops, how we can detect it at increasingly earlier ages, and what types of interventions are most effective."

Insel claimed that though there's been "unequivocal progress, much work needs to be done. Reauthorization will be critical for continuing this momentum and this stability over the IACC over the next three years."

Representative Pitts asked Insel about risk factors for autism.

Insel talked about longitudinal studies of exposures "that may increase risk." He was quick to add, "We also have increasing evidence for the importance of genetics as a risk factor. Perhaps 15 percent of children with a diagnosis of autism-spectrum disorder today have a genetic mutation. Many of these we didn't know about even six months ago. . . . Probably the most important area going forward is understanding how these genetic and environmental effects interact."

Insel then went on to describe how "exciting" it is that they may be able to diagnosis autism "before the second birthday." He was very hopeful about diagnosing as early as fourteen months.

Next, Insel talked about the needs of those "transitioning to adulthood." He said they haven't been really focused on this area before, but they've heard from the public, and now they know this is important because services aren't there for young adults.

Insel said that services being provided for those with autism aren't the same everywhere in the country, and he described the need for better services as something "urgent."

Rep. Pallone: "What kind of environmental factors are we talking about?"

Insel, talking about the twins study, said that the study showed more of the risk of autism is environmental. Then he digressed into talking about disorders that are "absolutely genetic" like fragile X. "There may be some, we don't really know the number, in which the disorder is really generated by environmental factors, yet to be determined. But there's a lot of research going on to try to track down what those could be. Much of the data that we have so far, and I think we're still in the early days on this, has been pointing to factors that impact second trimester, so prenatal or early postnatal factors in some cases. And there's a range of them that are coming particularly out of the UC Davis effort that's funded by NIH, EPA, and CDC. . . . One of the things they're looking at, not only the antidepressant study you've already mentioned, but there are questions about environmental exposures to certain kinds of chemicals in fertilizers, there are questions about medications . . . whether certain kinds of illnesses prenatally might predispose and be a risk factor. The bottom line is we still don't know. And we don't know of any factor that gives us more than a small amount of the risk that explains this increase."

An Ohio representative asked why autism was once a rare disorder, and now one in 110 children have it. "What were those kids being diagnosed with before?"

Insel, smiling broadly: "That's a good question. We don't know how many of these children were diagnosed with some other childhood disorder . . . One of the things that's changed over time is that you can now give a diagnosis of autism-spectrum disorder and have one of these other diagnoses. Prior to 1991, that was not an option. But it's still not clear that all of these children had something else. The question that we really need to grapple with is whether this a real increase or not. I think that most people that have been in this field, as I have for more than two decades, would say it's not simply changing diagnosis, not simply greater awareness, not simply ascertainment that's better, but that there is a true increase, as there is in asthma, type I diabetes, food allergies. There are more people affected with autism today than there were two decades ago. . . . Generally, children with autism become teenagers with autism, become adults with autism. They may adapt, they may be able to function better. Many of these children are able to go through a regular school system, but only with a great number of supports, often a very intensive and extensive set of behavioral therapies. The average cost estimate over lifetime is about $3.2 million per person on the spectrum."

A representative from Kentucky asked what we exactly know about autism.

Insel: "Go where we have the most traction, and, right now, that's in genetics. . . ."

Insel talked about the human genome study. But that's only going to explain part of the problem. He said they're looking into what could be the environmental factors that are affecting those people who are "genetically susceptible."

"As I was saying before, we have a very short list at this point because this is in some ways a relatively new area of investigation, and, to be honest about it, we don't have the traction in finding environmental factors that we do have in finding genetic sequence changes. So this is a long, expensive, and difficult process that mostly deals with large-population studies and goes after correlations, so it's not quite the same as we've been doing in genetics. That said, there are a number of projects underway. Some of which are looking at younger siblings . . . some are looking at large birth cohorts . . . some are looking in great detail at environmental factors that . . . uh . . . across both pregnancy and the first three years of life. All of those, when done longitudinally, may begin to flesh out some signals, but right now the signals we have are relatively weak. They may show, like with the antidepressants, perhaps a two-, maybe threefold increase in risk, but uh ... nothing like the seventyfold increase in risk that you have for having an identical twin."

Insel was asked about where he thinks all this is going, and he said we'll probably end up using "the power of genomics in actually finding environmental factors. . . . We may be able to find the footprints of environmental exposures by looking at the genome long after they take place. We're not there yet, but we're now getting the tools, and by 'now,' I mean in the last year or two, we have the tools to begin to do this with great precision and great throughput. And at that point, I think we'll be able to make a little more progress than we have to look for environmental causes."

Insel mentioned how inspired he is by autism parents. He was asked about the research at the Autism Centers of Excellence. This research "has been described by some as being redundant and too focused on genes and diagnosis research and not on ... things like autoimmune problems. In addition, there's concern that administrative costs are too high and that they take away much-needed funds from research."

Insel talked about the Eleven Autism Centers of Excellence. He claimed that these places are looking at environmental factors, especially long-term exposures. He praised the IACC for coordinating autism-research efforts.

Insel went on at length about what the term "autism-spectrum disorder" means. He talked about how it's lots of disorders "under this disorder."

One representative asked Insel about the "spectrum"—people who "may have gone through life always thought to be a little odd, but now they're actually diagnosed." This was followed by a question about the cost of $3.2 million. "Was this for someone with full-blown autism?"

Insel said, "Yes."

Insel was asked how many people with autism were going to cost this much to society. He couldn't give an answer at first but said 50 or 60 percent of those with autism fit that category. He also added that they "would have been identified twenty years ago because they don't have a subtle problem."

The next question was, "What is going to be the cost to society, and what is the potential of early intervention to diminish that cost?"

Insel talked about how important early intervention was. Then he made a stunning statement: "The cost to society which we've tried to model out in various ways ... I can tell you that the $3.2 million on average ...uh, you can multiply ...times... the 700,000 *people* who are on the spectrum, it's fair to say somewhere around that 500,000 are going to be on the severe end of the spectrum."

Next, one member thanked Dr. Insel for the work that IACC has done over the last decade.

Insel was again asked about the expenses of the Centers of Excellence and their expenditures. Insel talked about funding that involved hundreds of millions of dollars.

One congressman said, "There are those who say we're spending more for overhead than we're actually getting in research."

Insel said fifty percent of spending went for "overhead."

Insel finished by talking about the biology of autism and schizophrenia and about the "urgent need for medications" for autism. Finally, he focused on the "successes of the IACC." In the last minute and a half, he tossed out terms like sleep disorders and GI problems connected with autism "that are really quite common."

Next, it was announced, "That concludes our questioning for the panel, very excellent panel."

So what is going to happen when this disabled generation reaches adulthood if we're so uncertain about autism right now? We will be faced with providing for a never-ending population of disabled Americans that we can't explain. A significant portion of them will never be employable. We'll all be paying to support them. They will drain the financial resources of our society. We can't even imagine what autism is going to cost this nation. Twenty years from now, Americans caught in the autism nightmare will ask how things could possibly have gotten so bad, with authorities doing nothing to stop it. The abysmal inaction of those we call "experts" will be seen as outrageous and incomprehensible.

And as health officials and Congress for the most part muddle along scratching their heads over autism, the impact on the states has been undeniable. On April 28, 2009, President pro tem of the California State Senate Darrell Steinberg announced the establishment of the Senate Select Committee on Autism. Steinberg said that their intention was to make autism a "public health priority."[42] Unfortunately, Thomas Insel was not in attendance.

Various state officials and autism advocates spoke explaining what their work would include. They talked about the cost of autism, the need for services, and the shocking numbers in California.

While Steinberg made a reference to the "prevention of autism," no one expanded on this idea during the press conference. A number of upcoming bills were talked about.

One state senator aims to help with early diagnosing and intervention. Someone else is working on housing for people with autism. Another senator is focusing on employment for affected adults.

One speaker gave the mind-boggling California numbers, saying that there were "14,000 students with autism a decade ago." Then he added the increase: "46,000 students today, and growing."

Incredibly, no one at the press conference said, "We have to find out why this is happening to so many children. We can't keep adding thousands of children like this. This is a national health care emergency."

Rick Rollens of the MIND Institute spoke and made what I thought were the best comments. These were among the things he said:

> Autism is epidemic in this state as it is throughout the country.
>
> Autism population is skewed dramatically toward young children.
>
> Eighty-four percent of the autism population is under the age of twenty-one.
>
> More six- and seven-year-olds in the system than all the adults with autism combined.

What these people are talking about is reality. This is what autism is doing to our country. When Steinberg pointed out the billions of dollars autism is costing us now and the billions more autism will be costing as these kids age out into adulthood, no one made the claim that autism has always been around like this.

And no one said that these kids are going to outgrow autism because there is absolutely no evidence in the real world that it happens.

How long can we address autism by lighting the world up in blue lights and doing nothing about autism?

On April 2, 2013, Autism Awareness Day, the Secretary of Health and Human Services, Katherine Sebelius, issued a statement about autism: "During National Autism Awareness Month, we reflect on an urgent public health challenge and rededicate ourselves to addressing the complex needs of people with autism and their families. Over the last decade, we've learned that autism is far more prevalent than we had previously believed, affecting one out of every 110 American children. While we still have a lot to learn about what causes autism and which treatments can help people with autism thrive, we're getting closer to finding answers, thanks to a historic new investment in autism research . . ."[43]

Compare that to the message from HHS back in 2008, the first Autism Awareness Day/Month, Tuesday, April 1, 2008:

> Today, on the first World Autism Awareness Day, we pause to reaffirm our commitment to protecting the health of children in our country and throughout the world. Our determination remains strong as we continue our research efforts to increase understanding of how to treat and prevent autism and autism-spectrum disorders.
>
> People with these conditions and members of their families rely on the knowledge that science can offer. But there is much we do not yet understand. This is why we actively pursue research into genetic and environmental factors that may be involved in autism, and why we search for new treatments and therapies that may improve the quality of life for people with autism. Although we continue to evaluate vaccine safety to ensure we are providing the safest immunizations for our children, there is no credible scientific evidence to date that links vaccines to the development of autism, Therefore, we recommend that parents continue to have their children vaccinated. Vaccines have been one of the greatest medical advances in the past century. Vaccines have prevented—in some cases eliminated—many childhood diseases that were once considered unavoidable.
>
> We know that autism is a heart-wrenching condition that presents special challenges for many families. While we are physicians, we are also parents. We want parents of all children with autism to know that we are listening to them, not just today, but every day.[44]

Back in 2008, the statement was twice as long as in 2013, and it was a joint statement from the CDC, FDA, NIH, and HHS.

In 2008, the issue of a link between vaccines and autism was addressed with a strong denial and a recommendation to parents to vaccinate. In 2010, Sebelius didn't bring up the controversial topic.

In 2008, autism was described as "a heart-wrenching condition," but in 2010, Sebelius has reduced that to "an urgent public health challenge."

While the rate for autism in 2008 was one in every 150 children and by 2010, one in every 110, Sebelius, said only that "we've learned that autism is far more prevalent than we had previously believed."

In 2008, officials marked WAAD by saying they were looking for ways to "prevent autism." In 2010, Sebelius doesn't use the word "prevent."

In 2008, officials noted that they were actively pursuing "environmental factors" that may be involved in autism. By 2010, the word "environmental" isn't used when Sebelius mentioned autism research.

The one thing in common in both statements is the admission that health authorities can't tell us anything substantial about a disorder overwhelming a generation of children.

In 2008, the public was told, "There is much we do not yet understand." In 2010, Sebelius was still saying, "We still have a lot to learn about what causes autism."

Not a lot changed between 2008 and 2010 except that the severity of the autism epidemic seemed to be downplayed a bit more. And there was one other difference. In 2008, health officials promised: "We want parents of all children with autism to know that we are listening to them, not just today, but every day."

By 2010, Sebelius didn't even pretend any US health official was interested in what parents have to say.

In the real world, experts were looking at the numbers with growing concern. The argument that each and every increase in autism was due to doctors figuring out how to diagnose it made no sense. Where were the adults? Why were rate studies always done on children? Why was there no research on people in their forties and fifties?

On June 11, 2014, AltHealthWorks.com published an article that showed where this was all headed.[45]

Nick Meyer's title, "MIT Researcher's New Warning: At Today's Rate, Half of All US Children Will Be Autistic (by 2025)," might have seemed too far-fetched to be real to the ordinary reader. Surely, if things were really going to get this bad, the government would do something. Medical experts would be sounding an alarm. A rate so horrific might have been dismissed as merely impossible, idle speculation, an exaggeration with no basis in fact. To anyone actually reading the article, it didn't look that way. Meyer wrote, "Research scientist Stephanie Seneff, of the Massachusetts Institute of Technology (MIT), a widely published author on topics ranging from Azlheimer's Disease to autism and cardiovascular disease, raised plenty of eyebrows recently with a bold proclamation on autism at a special panel in Massachusetts about genetically modified organisms and other topics.

"'At today's rate, by 2025, one in two children will be autistic,' Seneff said last Thursday in Groton, Massachusetts, at an event sponsored by the holistic-focused Groton Wellness organization."

How could this be ignored? Dr. Seneff was from MIT—a leading US research university. Incredible at it seems, no mainstream news outlet covered her findings. No one was willing to explore the possibility that there is really something happening to the health of our children. This was also proof that the autism numbers are meaningless and that no one in the press takes them seriously at all.

# CHAPTER NINE
# ADMITTING THE TRUTH

*"Jim Adams predicts he'll have the final results of his study by the end of the year, and we'll have them first, here on* Dateline."

—John Larson, *NBC Dateline,* 2006

The controversy over a link between vaccines and autism shows no signs of going away. Despite lots of money spent on population studies at big-name universities conducted by well-credentialed experts, parents continue to be frightened by the potential for harm from the ever-expanding vaccine schedule recommended for all children, starting with the hepatitis B vaccine, given within hours of birth. Over the last two decades, the media has regularly reported on the latest study announced by the agency that runs the vaccine program, all showing no link between vaccines or components of vaccines and the development of autism. At the same time the public receives endless mixed messages about autism, the one tenet of faith at the Centers for Disease Control and Prevention has been that all the available science shows vaccines do not cause autism.

It's easy to understand why the claim persists. No one in mainstream medicine can reasonably explain why we have so many children with an autism diagnosis today. There's nothing a doctor can tell a new mother whose baby was born healthy and is developing normally so that her child doesn't also suddenly get sick, stop making eye contact and talking, lose learned skills, and regress into autism. When this happens, the only thing the doctor can be sure of is that the change had nothing to do with the battery of vaccination the child had received within hours, days, or weeks of this regression.

Other than their endless studies, the medical community has only guesses about autism—about every aspect of autism. No one is sure about an increase. News stories regularly assure us that all the autism is just better diagnosing on the part of doctors. Kids that used to be called "mentally retarded" or just "quirky" now fall in the autism category; it just *seems* like there's more autism. There have been endless stories about finding the genes or genetic mutations that cause a child to have autism. Whenever the rate is updated, the CDC can't tell how much, if any, is a true increase. And no one is ever alarmed. Autism is never a crisis in the minds of officials. Everything is under control. The disorder with no known cause or cure is nothing to worry about.

When the cause of autism is talked about, the subject of a link to vaccines inevitably comes up. Most of time, the topic is dismissed in a sentence or two. The press quickly informs the public that all the research out there has failed to show that vaccines are the cause of autism, that the single study by a British doctor in 1998 has been retracted, and that he lost his license to practice medicine in the UK. It's reassuring to hear this. No parent would want to think that the vaccines their child received had the potential to do this kind of damage. If news reports constantly present health officials, medical organizations, and the local pediatrician all saying the same thing, it must be true. It can't be the vaccines.

Coverage of things like the Pace Law School's "Unanswered Questions," Dr. Bernadine Healy, Hannah Poling, David Kirby's *Evidence of Harm*, and Robert Kennedy, Jr.'s "Deadly Immunity" are momentary ripples, and they quickly fade from the networks and the print news; once again we're told that there is no link and no possibility of a link. How is it that nothing is ever the smoking gun that finally forces major news outlets to concede that, at least for some children, vaccines are the trigger for autism?

The best way to answer that question is by example. In 2006, the NBC show *Dateline* covered the vaccine-autism controversy in a report called, "The Unorthodox Practice of Chelation."[1] NBC correspondent John Larson explored the possibility that children with autism are often unable to excrete toxic metals, especially mercury, and that removing the metals will improve their symptoms. His story was about Jim Adams, a professor of chemistry at Arizona State University, who was conducting a study to see if removing metals through chelation made a difference in their autism.

Larson: "Jim's suspicion that mercury might somehow be connected to the rise in the number of children diagnosed with autism places him near the center of one of the most hotly contested and politically charged medical debates of our time—one that has pitted activist parents against federal health officials and vaccine manufacturers, because mercury in children often comes from vaccines."

Larson acknowledged the toxicity of thimerosal. He said that, even though ethyl-mercury is different from methyl-mercury, in high enough doses, it can harm the nervous system.

It must have been more than a little concerning when Jim Adams then informed viewers that thimerosal was never tested or approved by the FDA. Since it was used in vaccines before the establishment of the agency, it was "just grandfathered in." More and more mercury-containing vaccines were added to the schedule during the 1990s, and it wasn't until 1999 that Congress asked the FDA to look into all the thimerosal in medical products.

The question from Larson: Was there a link between mercury-containing vaccines and autism?

To answer that question, Larson cited two studies from the CDC which exonerated vaccines with thimerosal as causal. He also talked with Tanja Popovic, CDC Associate Director for Science Research, on camera, who assured viewers, "Top-notch scientists have reviewed everything and anything that is available and have really in their latest report said that they reject causal association of thimerosal in vaccines and autism."

If that weren't enough to convince the audience that mainstream medicine disagreed with Jim Adams, Larson also included Dr. Jay Berkelhamer, president of the American Academy of Pediatrics, who said, "The usefulness of chelation therapy in treating autism is nil." Berkelhamer went on to describe the practice as "potentially toxic."

According to Larson, doctors were in agreement with the AAP that thimerosal doesn't cause autism. He added that experts say that kids may "outgrow the problem" or get better from therapy. What they didn't believe was that removing heavy metals had any affect on autism.

Jim Adams didn't accept that. In his mind, the science was still not conclusive on chelation.

Viewers were then told about a double-blind, placebo-controlled chelation study being conducted by Adams and Dr. Matt Boral of the Southwest College of Naturopathic Medicine—an accredited school of alternative and integrated medicine. The goal of the study was to determine if chelation can help children with autism.

Larson asked Adams about his potential bias in conducting such a study because his own daughter was autistic. Would that call his findings into question?

Incredibly, *Dateline* gave us people from the CDC and the AAP, two organizations with direct ties to the vaccination schedule, who, as expected, denied that mercury in vaccines is related to autism and that chelation is a factor in recovering affected kids—without a mention of what they have at stake in this debate.

Adams said he really had no choice but to conduct this study himself—no one else was willing to do research on chelating autistic children. Incredibly, he acknowledged that 23,000 families supported the practice of chelation for their children.

Regardless of results, Adams said that they would be made public.

To his credit, John Larson promised *Dateline* would follow up on the study. "Jim Adams predicts he'll have the final results of his study by the end of the year, and we'll have them first, here on *Dateline*."

In researching this topic, I was excited to see this kind of commitment from NBC, but, unfortunately, I was unable to find the *Dateline* coverage of results of the chelation study. I contacted Jim Adams at Arizona State and asked him what happened. Why didn't *Dateline* publish the results? His answer was brief: "*Dateline* was not interested in following up at that time."

In the original *Dateline* story, they acknowledged that the autism rate that was "only one in 10,000 children in the 1980s was two decades later diagnosed in as many as one in every 175 American children," and, yet, they offered no explanation. Why not tell us if this chelation therapy might offer some hope or if it wasn't worth pursuing?

I looked at the results of Adams' study, which seemed to show that chelating this test group was both safe and beneficial. I asked him to summarize the effects of the therapy.

He wrote me,

> We found that DMSA therapy, using our schedule, was very safe and generally well-tolerated.
>
> It was effective in reducing toxic metals from children, especially lead. Roughly 20 percent of children did not have significant levels of urinary excretion, roughly 20

> percent needed treatment for one to two months, and 60 percent needed treatment for longer than three months (the study was limited to three months). There were significant improvements in autism symptoms, and the degree of improvement correlated with the amount of toxic metals excreted—i.e., those with more excretion of toxic metals generally had more improvement.
>
> A surprise of the study was that one round of DMSA therapy normalized glutathione, the body's primary antioxidant and defense against toxic metals. This may explain why one round of DMSA therapy led to almost as much improvement as seven rounds; a simple analogy is that if one aspirin is enough to cure a headache, then seven aspirin is not necessarily better.
>
> In terms of safety, there was a small increase in excretion of potassium and chromium, but that is easily countered by eating a serving of fruit or vegetables and taking a multivitamin/mineral supplement that includes chromium.
>
> Since the results of the study were very promising, it should be followed up with a randomized, double-blind, placebo-controlled study to confirm the results.
>
> Based on these results, I think every child with autism should try a single dose of DMSA (10 mg/kg bodyweight) and measure urinary excretion of toxic metals before the DMSA and for six to eight hours after. If there is a significant excretion of toxic metals (above the lab's reference range), then I think they should continue DMSA therapy until those levels are decreased, while also trying to limit exposure to toxic metals.

Like Wakefield before him, Adams didn't say he had proof that vaccines cause autism. He simply asked for more research, just like Wakefield. No one seemed willing to do that. They didn't want to ask questions about toxins and autism. The implications were too great.

Mounting evidence linking vaccines to the epidemic rise in autism coincided with a shocking admission from Health and Human Services Secretary Kathleen Sebelius in *Reader's Digest*, also in March 2010.[2] In an interview by Arthur Allen on the H1N1 vaccine, Sebelius was asked the general question, "What can be done about public mistrust of vaccines?"

Her answer had far-reaching implications.

Sebelius: "There are groups out there that insist that vaccines are responsible for a variety of problems, despite all scientific evidence to the contrary. We have reached out to media outlets to try to get them to not give the views of these people equal weight in their reporting to what science has shown and continues to show about the safety of vaccines."

Was autism among the "variety of problems" linked to vaccines? What right did a government official have in asking news sources to censor unfavorable opinion on vaccines? Sebelius was well aware that medical experts in her department had conceded the vaccine-injury case of Hannah Poling. Nothing more was done to determine how many other children had the same mitochondrial predisposition that linked her vaccinations to her autism. How willing were members of the press to comply with pressure from HHS?

April 27, 2010, PBS ran the *Frontline* story "The Vaccine War," which purported to examine "the emotionally charged debate over medical risks vs. benefits and a parent's right to make choices about her child vs. a community's common good."[3]

The very title was misleading. The word "war" makes one think of a conflict with two sides. That's not what PBS presented to the public, however, and anyone with even a rudimentary under-standing of the vaccine controversy could recognize the spin.

On their website, PBS promoted this show saying, "In 'The Vaccine War,' *Frontline* lays bare the science of vaccine safety and examines the increasingly bitter debate between the public health establishment and a formidable populist coalition of parents, celebrities, politicians, and activists who are armed with the latest social media tools—including Facebook, YouTube, and Twitter—and are determined to resist pressure from the medical and public health establishments to vaccinate, despite established scientific consensus about vaccine safety."

In truth, what viewers witnessed on PBS was yet another example of media bias and a distorted reporting of the facts. Parents have grown weary of the mantra "Vaccines are safe, vaccines save lives." How many times has this issue been declared settled? How many studies have been announced showing vaccines don't have serious side effects like autism? This debate shows no signs of stopping, despite the ardent efforts of shows like *Frontline*.

The claims of parents were noted and dismissed by *Frontline*. PBS portrayed parents as impassioned and determined but totally without any science on their side. Jenny McCarthy, JB Handley, Barbara Loe Fisher, and Robert Kennedy, Jr., along with a number of non-vaccinating parents, were included. To the general public, the message was clear: The medical community is solidly lined up against such parents. The anti-vaccine movement is based on fraudulent research (Andrew Wakefield) and celebrity leadership (Jenny McCarthy).

So why do the show?

Why give more publicity to the phony claim that vaccines have harmful side effects?

Maybe the answer is that despite the best efforts of health officials and their willing followers in the media, the public isn't buying it. Parents are scared. Autistic children are everywhere in our schools, and no one can reasonably explain where they're all coming from. A lot of the *Frontline* show was about the power of the Internet. Offit declared that people are getting phony information from watching YouTube videos. The Internet is the dangerous influence, according to all these health experts. Fisher, McCarthy, and Handley use this forum to influence the public. Parents are exempting their children, and we're losing herd immunity. This is becoming a national health threat.

There was nothing new in what the pro-vaccine people had to say. We were reminded that they're focused on saving lives. Nothing was new from the other side, either. Parents continue to hang on to the false belief that vaccines can harm children. It's hard to imagine what PBS hoped to accomplish with this show.

What we never hear:

Notice that under no circumstance does anyone ever bring up what else motivates the medical community and health officials. No one mentions that these people have everything at stake in this debate. If countless parents are right, and vaccines *have* damaged a generation of children, people will be held responsible—the same people who tell us vaccines are safe. Media sources like PBS like to pretend that this is just about the science, but any clear-thinking person knows that's not the case.

There was another element missing from the PBS coverage. Where were the experts on our side? Why did PBS make it seem that only parents are concerned about vaccine safety? Did they make any effort to find any of the well-credentialed scientists and doctors who disagree with the mainstream medical community?

The answer is "Yes"—they found them two of them. PBS interviewed Jay Gordon, MD, and Robert Sears, MD. They discussed the issue with producer Kate McMahon for several hours each.

Gordon is a nationally renowned pediatrician and Assistant Professor of Pediatrics, UCLA Medical School.

Sears is also well known and the author of several books, including ones on vaccines and on autism.

So what happened to their interviews?

McMahon said Gordon was cut because it was "best for the show." I spoke with Dr. Sears, and he said that he was told that his interview was cut because "there was too much footage." Paul Offit was shown a number of times on the broadcast, but there wasn't thirty seconds for either Sears or Gordon.

Sears's interview was on the PBS website; Gordon's was not.

Sears made it clear that he's pro-vaccine. He hoped that by offering an alternative schedule, reluctant parents will continue to vaccinate their children.

He's hardly the threat to herd immunity that non-vaccinating parents are, but incredibly, *Frontline* made no mention of Dr. Sears.

The only way the story presented by *Frontline* works is if we just forget about autism. We have to pretend that there's been no real increase. The vaccine schedule may be more than three times what it was in 1983, but it hasn't caused any problems. The only epidemics we need to worry about are the ones caused by non-vaccinating parents.

The real problem is that autism isn't going away. We're talking about hundreds of thousands of affected children who will live long lives, many severely disabled and totally dependent. PBS may try to change the subject and ignore the reality of what's happened to our children, but the public hears more and more about autism every day in the news. As these affected children age into adulthood, they will cost billions of dollars each year for their support and care, and their numbers will be replaced by another generation of children. This is the scariest scenario I can imagine. And no one is talking about it.

Among the questions Bob Sears was asked were these two: "What if vaccines turn out to be a red herring? What if we're so off the mark with vaccines?"

Kate McMahon should have asked him two more questions: What if vaccines turn out to be the cause of the autism epidemic? What if all those questioning vaccine safety are right?

The *New York Times* wrote about *"The Vaccine War"* in a supportive piece entitled, *"Vaccinations: A Hot Debate Still Burning"* by Neil Genzlinger.[4] The *Times* dismissed the idea that vaccines were a risk, citing Jenny McCarthy and Jim Carrey, "who are concerned that vaccines cause harm; scientific studies from around the world find that they don't."

According to the *Times*, unbelieving parents were merely indulging in conspiracy theories that threatened the herd immunity of us all.

On April 28, 2010, Jenny McCarthy posted her reaction to the *Frontline* coverage on *Huffington*:

"When the producers of PBS's *Frontline* approached me to be interviewed for their new documentary 'The Vaccine War,' I accepted with a simple condition: Doctors and scientists on our side of the vaccine-autism debate needed to have a voice, too.

"Prior to agreeing to the interview, Frontline sent us this email:

"'*Frontline* will carry out a detailed and even-handed investigation, including voices from all sides of the controversy, including parents, activists, physicians, scientists, lawyers, politicians and vaccine manufacturers.'"[5]

According to McCarthy, she was tired of how the media presents this as a debate between parents and medical experts. When *Frontline* asked her to do the interview, she insisted that Los Angeles pediatrician Jay Gordon be included.

McCarthy said *Frontline* "broke their promise." They "presented our entire community's position through my interview and just two other parents—Barbara Loe Fisher and J. B. Handley."

This is typical of how the media covers autism and vaccines. McCarthy asked, "Where are the doctors and scientists who support our community and support the idea that vaccines may be a trigger for autism? In *Frontline's* world, they don't exist."

Even a veteran journalist can fail us. Bill Moyers, who once served as press secretary for President Lyndon Johnson and worked for Newsday, NBC and PBS, wrote the *Counterpunch* story "When the Next Contagion Strikes—Vaccination Nation," with Michael Winship on March 1, 2012.[6] It was a review of the movie *Contagion*, about the spread of a global pandemic. Moyers and Winship expanded on the theme of the movie and speculated on the possibility that it could happen here: "Rarely does a film issue such an inescapable invitation to think: 'It could happen; that could be us.' What would we do?"

The rest of the piece was about the importance of vaccines and the dangers we all face because some parents are too afraid of autism to vaccinate their children. According to the writers, "science has largely debunked" any link between vaccines and autism. They were satisfied with the findings of the official studies without asking who funded the study or who did the research, and they never considered that there might be science on the other side.

I was first aware of autism mom Alison MacNeil when I watched the PBS series "Autism Now," in 2011.[7] On April 18, 2011, Alison's father, veteran journalist Robert MacNeil, hosted the first of a six-part series on autism. During the show, MacNeil focused on his grandson with autism. MacNeil said, "In recent years, the diagnosis of autism has shown startling growth, now affecting one in 110 American children. For over two decades, parents desperate for answers and feeling slighted by the medical community have felt forced to create services for their children, raise money for research, and to campaign for wider awareness for autism and for support from the government." He continued, telling viewers about the genetic research going on, and he noted the possibility that "toxic ingredients in the environment may trigger the symptoms of autism."

MacNeil explained that his six-year-old grandson Nick lived in Cambridge, Massachusetts, and that this was the first time in his fifty years as a journalist that he'd ever included a family member in anything that he'd covered. Viewers were shown a photo of MacNeil holding a smiling baby, and he said, "This was Nick when he was nine months old, a healthy, alert, engaged baby with no apparent medical problems."

MacNeil was shown visiting with Nick and his family. He said that his grandson at six was "like a different child, showing the classic symptoms of autism." MacNeil described Nick's rigid, withdrawn behavior as "relatively mild" autism.

The audience heard that Nick has health issues along with his autism, including seizures, sensory, mitochondria, and gut problems. MacNeil said that Nick's condition was "devastating" to his daughter Alison. The camera covered Alison and her father sitting on the couch as Alison talked about how Nick started spinning plates when he was sixteen months old—a classic sign of autism. Nick also wouldn't respond to his mother's voice. Following this, a developmental pediatrician diagnosed him with autism.

Something had happened to Nick just before this change in his behavior. His mother said, "We went from a fifteen-month appointment where this child was A-okay, supposedly, and given the MMR, the DTap, and the Hib vaccines."

Alison said that people told her that this was just a coincidence. She wasn't buying that—"his whole system shut down. Something happened to my child."

Robert MacNeil immediately said that health officials denied any connection because there was no science backing the claim that vaccines cause autism.

Alison got little help from doctors. She described going to the doctor about her son's chronic diarrhea, a condition he endured for months following his fifteen-months vaccines.

Her pediatrician was unconcerned. Alison said she was told that diarrhea is something that is common for children with autism and that all of Nick's symptoms were just "part of autism."

Nick's gastroenterologist had a view at odds with the pediatrician's. He described the damage to Nick's GI tract and said that when a child reacts to this gut pain with changes in sleep and behavior, it's often dismissed as just part of autism, and the real cause is ignored.

Robert MacNeil brought up the failure of the medical community to deal with the autism crisis when he asked his daughter if she believed doctors understood all the issues involved in autism.

Alison was adamant that the medical community was not doing enough for children with autism. She said they weren't addressing GI problems or looking for signs of seizure activity.

MacNeil talked about the incredible toll that Nick's autism has taken on every member of his family, including his ten-year-old sister, Neely. Neely was part of the interview, and she talked about all of Nick's special needs and her worries about his care in the future.

Nick's distress over a change in his schedule was shown. This is how autism affects even the higher-functioning kids. MacNeil said that Nick's ability to disassociate himself from his surroundings and lose eye contact caused him pain personally.

As part of the "Autism Now" series, there was also an interview with Dr. David Amaral, a leading autism researcher at the MIND Institute at the University of California at Davis. Robert MacNeil asked Dr. Amaral asked if vaccines can cause autism.

Amaral was cautious in his answer, saying, "I think it's pretty clear that, in general, vaccines are not the culprit." He cited the population studies and made the strange claim that children who are fully vaccinated "are at slightly less risk of having autism than children that aren't immunized."

What followed was a truly amazing admission from someone in his position.

While Amaral didn't believe that vaccines were "a major cause of autism," he added: "It's not to say, however, that there isn't a small subset of children who may be particularly vulnerable to vaccines.

"And in their case, having the vaccines, or particular vaccines, particularly in certain kinds of situations—if the child was ill, if the child had a precondition, like a mitochondrial defect. Vaccinations for those children actually may be the environmental factor that tipped them over the edge of autism."

Amaral said there should be research looking at "vulnerabilities" in certain children that "might make them at risk for having certain vaccinations."

It sounded like Amaral covered all his bases. He denied a link between vaccines and the development of autism. In fact, he said vaccinated kids were "at slightly less risk of having autism." Then he said vaccines weren't "a major cause of autism." Finally, he called for more research into whether or not a vulnerable group may be at risk for autism if they're vaccinated.

This part of the "Autism Now" series was on April 20, 2011, two days after the segment where Robert MacNeil's daughter said that the series of vaccinations her son received at his fifteen-month check-up caused an immediate change in his health and behavior and led to his regression into autism. Did MacNeil wonder if his grandson was one of the "small subset of children" that David Amaral talked about? Now, three years after the 2011 PBS series, nothing more has been done about researching who these at-risk kids might be. The MIND Institute never followed up on the science that Amaral said was "incredibly important" back in 2011.

In July, 2012, I wrote a piece for *Age of Autism* about the efforts of a mother with a severely affected autistic child to reach out to the media.[8] "The Truth About Liz Szabo and *USA Today* RE Autism Coverage" was all about how one reporter refused to concede that there might be two sides to the autism-vaccine controversy. *USA Today* medical reporter Liz Szabo is someone who has long downplayed what autism is doing to our children. She's especially adamant that vaccines aren't a factor. She's done such a good job promoting the claim that studies show no link that vaccine developer Dr. Paul Offit personally thanked her in his book *Deadly Choices.*

Szabo had a piece in *USA Today* on April 2, 2012, called "With autism rising, researchers step up hunt for a cause."[9] There was nothing new in the piece. She cited possible contributing factors, including genes, prematurity, low birth weight, medications, and having babies too close together. Readers were reminded that vaccines were not involved. "Doctors can reassure parents that one thing doesn't cause autism: vaccines, says Paul Offit, chief of infectious diseases at Children's Hospital of Philadelphia. Nearly two dozen studies have failed to find a link between autism and vaccines, whether given alone or in combination."

In truth, there's more to Szabo's April 2, 2012, story, and it reveals a lot about the mindset of many reporters in the mainstream press. The mother of a seven-year-old boy with severe autism talked to me about a meeting she had with Szabo just before her April 2 story was published. Jackie Murphy of South San Francisco was asked by the MIND Institute at UC-Davis to be interviewed by Szabo for her story. Murphy, whose son Fintan had participated in studies at the MIND, wanted to do more than just talk to Szabo on the phone. She actually flew to Washington, DC, at her own expense so she could share her son's medical records with Szabo. She talked to her for more than two hours, presenting her son's medical history and what she understood about her son's autism from her perspective as a registered nurse. Murphy tried to get Szabo to consider that there are actually two sides to this controversy. Murphy brought her son's detailed medical files and even provided a picture of the large gastrointestinal ulcer her son had at age two and a half. She thought that this would be compelling enough to motivate Szabo to look into the serious immune system/GI system problems common in autistic children.

Murphy told Szabo what she observed when her son was vaccinated. Fintan received six vaccines when he was two, at a time when he was recovering from an upper-respiratory-tract infection and severe anemia, conditions of which his doctor was aware. Her son, who was already having problems, became extremely ill and lost all ability to communicate. She told Szabo that to this day Fintan has almost no expressive language and no understanding of what's being said to him.

Murphy hoped this would make a difference. She knew that children like Fintan are everywhere and that reporters need to talk about them. Despite all her efforts, nothing about her interview with Szabo appeared in the story. There was no mention of GI issues and regressive autism. Instead, parents were told specifically that there was no link to vaccines, and Thomas Insel, director of the National Institutes of Mental Health, was quoted saying, "In large part, the causes of autism . . . remain a mystery."

On May 1, 2013, the *Columbia University Journalism Review* published the piece "Sticking with the truth—How 'balanced' coverage helped sustain the bogus claim that childhood vaccines can cause autism," by Curtis Brainard.[10]

According to Brainard, media sources covering the controversy were "squandering journalistic resources on a bogus story." And not only that, "there is evidence that fear of a link between vaccines and autism, stoked by press coverage, caused some parents to either delay vaccinations for their children or decline them altogether."

What seemed most disturbing to Brainard was the fact that this subject just won't go away. He said that reporters have been waiting for this controversy to go away. It was clear to him that the reason this nagging theory is still around has got to be because the media continues to cover it:

> "Concern about adverse events, particularly related to media reports of a putative association between vaccinations and autism and of the dangers of thimerosal, appeared to play a major role in the decision of these families to decline vaccination," according to a 2006 study published in *The New England Journal of Medicine*.

Brainard seemed baffled that the public continues to doubt the safety claims. He cited the 2001 and 2004 studies by the Institute of Medicine that debunked any kind of connections between vaccines and autism. The reason why the controversy lingers on must be because the press keeps bringing it up. Brainard cited Robert Kennedy, Jr.'s "Deadly Immunity" along with other examples. He was especially upset by what David Kirby and Dan Olmsted have written. According to Brainard, Kirby had presented "parental suspicions" that there was a link, and Olmsted had conducted a survey of parents for his series *Age of Autism* that showed "lower autism rates among ostensibly unvaccinated Amish communities."

Members of Congress have been convinced to look into the link, and notables like Jenny McCarthy have hopped on the anti-vaccine bandwagon, according to Brainard.

After reading this, I looked at the mission statement at his publication:

"*Columbia Journalism Review's* mission is to encourage excellence in journalism in the service of a free society." *CJR* "monitors and supports the press as it works across all platforms, and also tracks the ongoing evolution of the media business," and they "host a conversation that is open to all who share a commitment to high journalistic standards in the US and around the world."

Do those high journalistic standards include blindly trusting health officials and medical journals? Did Brainard ever once consider that citing studies and claims from the agency that runs the vaccine program isn't real proof of anything? Was Brainard aware that hundreds of individuals at the CDC have conflict-of-interest waivers because they have financial ties to the vaccine makers? Did he know that the last head of the CDC, Dr. Julie Gerberding, a long-time denier of any link, is now the head of the vaccine division at Merck?

Brainard needed to ask himself why study after official study showing no association between vaccines and autism have not been able to settle the question.

Brainard attacked David Kirby and Dan Olmsted and cited their writing but didn't say he'd actually read either *Evidence of Harm* or *The Age of Autism.* I wondered if he's ever looked at Wakefield's book *Callous Disregard.*

Brainard talked about the MMR vaccine and thimerosal-containing ones but made no mention of the fact that there were never adequate trials of the combined MMR vaccine and that no studies were ever done on thimerosal before it was allowed in vaccines.

He didn't bring up the fact that the British government indemnified the manufacturer of the MMR vaccine and that, therefore, it's the government that would be liable for damage resulting from this vaccine if a link were clearly recognized.

In Brainard's selective coverage, nothing was said about Hannah Poling, the Georgia girl whose vaccine-autism injury case was conceded by medical experts from HHS, nor did we hear about the dozens of other vaccine-injury cases involving autism that were compensated by the federal Vaccine Court and covered in the *Pace University Law Review* story "Unanswered Questions."

May 8, 2013, a journalism publication at MIT endorsed the view that the press wasn't obligated to cover both sides in the vaccine controversy and praised the Brainard article.[11] In the MIT piece, Deborah Blum wrote, "The strength of Brainard's piece, though, is that he pulls so much of this coverage together and in doing so demonstrates the destructive pattern. It's a warning against the problem of false balance in science reporting. And it's a reminder that we could do a whole lot better."

"Fair and balanced" no longer applies when the subject was vaccines and autism. To parents in the autism community, this was not news.

Pressure on journalists not to present both sides continued. On March 29, 2014, *Forbes* published an article entitled "Dr. Paul Offit:

'Journalism Jail' for Faulty Medical Reporting."[12] It was by David Kroll, who was described on the sidebar of the article as a pharmacologist and someone who teaches science and health writing and reporting courses. He added the disclaimer: "The views expressed here are mine alone and do not represent any official position of my employer or affiliated agencies."

The subject of this story was downright shocking to many readers. Kroll's piece was about the keynote speech by Dr. Offit at the annual meeting of the Association for Health Care Journalists (AHCJ) that was held in Denver, March 27 to March 30. Kroll wrote that Offit "called on broadcast and print reporters to avoid the 'he-said, she-said reporting' that perpetuates false controversies in science and medicine."

"False controversies"?

Offit's purpose was to caution members of the media that there really weren't two sides to the controversy over vaccine safety and that they were not obligated to cover it in a fair and balanced manner. Kroll referred to reporting on a link between vaccines and autism as "faulty." Offit was described as "troubled" by stories where journalists had "balance" in their reporting. According to Offit, too often he found himself forced to comment on what people like Donald Trump or Kristin Cavallari had to say about autism and vaccines. Kroll said Offit was qualified to speak on the subject because he was an expert, and these others were not. Offit objected to reporters including people who "don't know the data." He acknowledged that while vaccines do have side effects, "these side effects have absolutely nothing to do with causes invoked by many anti-vaccination activists."

Offit went even further during the question-and-answer session. Instead of anyone from the media challenging Offit's blanket rejection of any science supporting the link between vaccines and autism, one reporter asked if, when stories on the vaccine controversy caused parents not to vaccinate, would journalists be "party to murder?" Offit's flippant response was to say there should be "journalism jail" for anyone guilty of this.

This story from *Forbes* generated hundreds of responses in the comment section, and it was troubling in many ways. First of all, unlike almost all coverage of Paul Offit, Kroll started off by saying Offit was a "vaccine developer." Later in the story, he acknowledged how much Offit has personally profited from his work. "Offit himself is best known for his work in the 1980s that led to the development of a rotavirus vaccine, RotaTeq, licensed to Merck in 1992 by CHOP and The Wistar Institute. In 2008, CHOP sold their worldwide rights to royalties from the vaccine for $182 million. Offit's personal or laboratory share has never been disclosed publicly, but typical intellectual-property agreements in academic research allow for the inventors to share in up to 25 percent of institutional income."

The caption on a photo of Offit and RotaTeq co-inventor H. Fred Clark said: "Rotavirus vaccine inventor Paul Offit . . . routinely endures vitriolic attacks on his credibility, along with death threats, for defending the safety of vaccines."

Offit's overwhelming conflict of interest has no place in this debate, according to David Kroll. It seemed only to enhance his qualifications as "a highly-trained and experienced professional."

The whole idea of someone with strong industry ties as the keynote speaker at a conference of health care journalists is frightening. Coverage of the question-and-answers session that followed didn't include anyone who disagreed with Offit's call for censorship. What was amazing to us in the autism community was the whole idea that there is anything even approaching legitimate coverage of the autism-vaccine debate. No reporter mentions the independent science by top people that calls everything Offit said into question. No one ever asks about the industry ties of those promoting vaccines as safe, and it's clear from this piece that the conflicts don't really matter to those writing on this topic. Stories supposedly covering both sides in the debate most of time cite "experts" like Offit and people like Jenny McCarthy and Dr. Andrew Wakefield. McCarthy is described as a "former *Playboy* bunny" and Wakefield as merely "a doctor who was found guilty of fraud." How much more unfair and unbalanced could it get? According to Offit, even citing anyone who links vaccines to autism is unacceptable and needs to stop. The public should only hear one thing about vaccines—vaccines are safe, vaccines save lives.

The reporters at this conference were told how to do their job by someone who's spent years vilifying anyone sounding an alarm over vaccine side effects and the epidemic increase in autism. This has far-reaching effects. Members of the media overwhelmingly report each stunning worsening of the autism rate as no real increase and no real crisis. If autism isn't a problem, then we don't have to be really worried about the cause. Given this atmosphere, there's no need to bring up the subject of vaccines.

Those who need to cover up how bad the autism epidemic really is, along with all evidence of the vaccine link, need the media to be totally onboard. Members of the press have to understand that any coverage of the other side, can't be tolerated. The veiled threat that parents not vaccinating and children getting sick will be reporters' fault is an added element. The only job of health reporters is to promote vaccines as safe and effective. Anything else is not to be tolerated and may even be criminal.

According to their website, the Association for Health Care Journalists is an "independent, nonprofit organization dedicated to advancing public understanding of health care issues. Its mission is to improve the quality, accuracy and visibility of health care reporting, writing and editing."[13]

So how does what Offit said fit into their stated goals of supporting "the highest standards of reporting, editing, and broadcasting in health care journalism"? The AHCJ also stated that their purpose was "to advocate for the free flow of information to the public," yet what Offit was calling for was the exact opposite of that.

Taking their marching orders from people like Offit should clearly violate their goals of raising the image of health care journalism and serving the public. Does advocating for "the free flow of information to the public" mean only the information approved by vaccine promoters like Paul Offit?

The media's determination to vilify anyone who dared suggest that vaccines and autism were linked intensified in April 2014. It came to light that the restaurant chain Chili's was going to donate 10 percent of its proceeds on April 7 to the National Autism Association. Immediately, the media went on the attack, accusing Chili's of supporting a group they said was "anti-vaccine."

Emily Willingham, at *Forbes,* wrote, "Chili's had made a particularly poor choice" in deciding to give money to NAA.[14] Willingham quoted their website:

"While mainstream science discounts vaccinations as a cause, members of the National Autism Association feel vaccinations have triggered autism in a subset of children, and that an overly aggressive vaccination schedule coupled with toxic adjuvants in vaccines could affect individuals who have a family history of autoimmune disorders specifically."

Willingham acknowledged the fact that there are parents who believe that vaccines triggered autism in their children hardly makes the NAA an anti-vaccine group, but according to Willingham, it didn't matter. She took issue with the fact that the NAA states the following on its website: "Vaccinations can trigger or exacerbate autism in some, if not many, children, especially those who are genetically predisposed to immune, autoimmune or inflammatory conditions.

"Other environmental exposures may trigger, or exacerbate, autism in certain children, especially those who are genetically predisposed to immune, autoimmune or inflammatory conditions."

Willingham didn't agree that there were any "environmental exposures" that were found to be linked to autism. "Their list consists of factors that have been correlated with autism risk, not established as causative or contributing, with some more compelling than others."

The *Forbes* article noted that it had been first posted at 8:10 PDT on April 6, and, at 2:30 PDT, Willingham added an update to her story. She said that she had received a statement from Chili's announcing that they were canceling Monday's Give Back Event because of "the feedback we heard from our guests." Chili's was going to find some other way of supporting children with autism.

It says a lot about *Forbes'* influence that Brinker International, the parent company of Chili's, would notify Willingham personally about their decision. It makes one wonder if the decision was based on "feedback . . . from our guests" or pressure from news sites like *Forbes*.

The National Autism Association ceased being an advocacy group for parents with disabled children. According to hundreds of news reports, the NAA was merely "an anti-vaccine charity."

The *Los Angeles Times* reported, "The National Autism Assn. promotes that nonexistent linkage. Its 'Causes of Autism' webpage states its belief that 'vaccines can trigger or exacerbate autism in some, if not many, children.' It adds, 'though published mainstream science fails to acknowledge a causal link' to vaccines and other 'environmental' causes, 'it's important that parental accounts be carefully considered.'"15 The *Times* said that what the NAA had up was "destructive" to "the health of children," and that statements like theirs were behind the measles outbreaks in California and elsewhere.

According to the *LA Times*, the very fact that the NAA mentioned that there are parents out there who believe vaccines caused their children's autism makes them a dangerous organization.

In their coverage of the Chili's story, *ABC News* said that, in addition to linking vaccines to autism, the National Autism Association was also guilty of promoting the use of chelation on their site.[16] Removing heavy metals as a treatment for autism is "unfounded and illogical," according to a 2013 study cited by *ABC News*.

Incredibly, almost none of the endless reports about Chili's and the NAA's position on vaccines mentioned that the proceeds were earmarked to be used for the NAA's efforts to protect autistic children from wandering. This is an especially critical work since the leading cause of death among those with autism is drowning.

Of all the media coverage of this, *TIME Magazine* was the worst.[17] On April 7, an opinion piece by Jeffrey Kluger appeared on *Google News* with the title "Chili's Burns Anti-Vaxxers: That's What Happens When You Kill and Maim Kids." It seemed that it wasn't enough to label the members of the NAA as "anti-vaccine"; *TIME* was also calling them murderers. I'm sure TIME must have had a lot of response after publishing a headline that sounded like tabloid rhetoric, at best—short on content, long on sensationalism, because within a couple of hours, it was replaced with "Chili's Burns Anti-Vaxxers—and Probably Saves Some Kids' Lives." Kluger called the NAA "anti-vaccine kooks" and added that the National Vaccine Information Center was "far more odious."

Since the vast majority of reporters do no investigation before they make their pronouncements about autism, there is absolutely no mention of the fact that in February 2012, Autism Speaks, the world's largest autism advocacy organization, announced that it awarded $30,000 to the National Autism Association in order to provide 1,000 of their "Big Red Safety Boxes" to families of children who were at risk for wandering.[18]

Autism Speaks vice president of Family Services Lisa Goring was quoted saying, "The National Autism Association has taken on a leadership role in raising awareness about the dangers of wandering and elopement for some individuals with autism. NAA's Big Red Safety Boxes provide the necessary resources to help prevent potentially dangerous situations, and we are proud to partner with the NAA to fund more of these valuable tools for families across the country."

It's hard to understand why a similar action by Chili's provoked such outrage from the media. Why didn't Emily Willingham call on Autism Speaks to reconsider their actions in 2012? Why didn't the *LA Times* criticize Autism Speaks like they did Chili's?

No matter, none of this factored into the media's overall condemnation of the National Autism Association. The message to any business wanting to donate to an autism group? make sure they don't support the claim of a link between vaccines and autism. The message to autism groups was also clear: You can hold walks for awareness and light things up in blue each April, but you're not allowed to bring up the cause—if it has anything to do with vaccines. Maybe the big difference between the fact no one attacked Autism Speaks in 2012 and the vendetta against Chili's in 2014 is the issue of vaccine safety. The claim that vaccines have serious side effects, including autism, can't be stamped out, no matter how many well-credentialed experts appear on network news shows or are covered in the *New York Times* saying there is no link. By 2014, it was time to stamp out any opposition and use the media to do it. The fact that Paul Offit was the keynote speaker at the Association for Health Care Journalists, advising them not to give balanced coverage to those worried about vaccine side effects in March 2014 and that, in April, major news outlets expressed their outrage that a restaurant chain would donate money to "an anti-vaccine" organization seemed to show that members of the media had their marching orders and that they were following them.

On April 28, 2014, Paul Offit appeared on Comedy Central's *the Colbert Report* and Stephen Colbert tried to turn vaccine-exempting parents into satirical comedy.[19]

In the six-and-a-half-minute interview with Offit, Colbert ignored the fact that officials are clueless when it comes to what causes autism—all that mattered was ridiculing anyone who dares to say it's linked to vaccines.

Amid all the sarcasm and kidding around, Offit described the lifesaving benefits of our ever-increasing vaccine schedule. He referenced twenty studies showing no link between vaccines and autism. The increase in the schedule and the explosion in autism was just a coincidence.

Colbert talked about thimerosal. He even said it's made from mercury. Viewers were shown an image of the skull and crossbones on the thimerosal container, which hardly seem to fit the claim that this stuff was supposed to be safe enough to inject into children and pregnant women.

Colbert said 29 percent of Americans don't believe Paul Offit. They think vaccines do cause autism. Celebrities and parents were the only ones who link the two, according to Colbert.

Colbert forgot to mention that Offit has financial ties to pharma. He never told the audience that vaccine makers have no liability. Likewise, no matter how sick a child gets from a vaccination, doctors are protected from any lawsuits.

Offit: "It's perfectly reasonable for the parent to ask the question." If their child was vaccinated and "now they aren't fine," they might assume there was some connection, but there really wasn't. According to Offit, it had been studied endlessly, and there never was any link proven. "The question is, Why does the 29 percent still think vaccines may be a problem when, in fact, they've been shown not to be?"

"Now they aren't fine" hardly describes what many children have experienced following vaccinations, including seizures, chronic diarrhea, sleep disorders, and loss of learned skills, including the ability to speak.

Colbert noted that Offit is the head of the Vaccine Education Center at the Children's Hospital of Philadelphia, and he asked him why we still needed to be educated.

Offit couldn't explain why parents weren't buying the safety claims. They should know by now that vaccines are safe.

Offit's ties to industry were acknowledged when Colbert asked him, "What if I were to tell you, you sound like you're in the pocket of Big Pharma."

Laughter and applause followed, but there was no mention of his work for Merck.

Paul Offit must love coming on shows like *The Colbert Report.* There was no pretense of balance here. Colbert and Offit have to hope that most people really are ignorant about this issue.

They're betting that viewers are impressed with an expert from CHOP who only wants to protect kids from dangerous diseases and that they have no idea that there are now hundreds of peer-reviewed studies by well-credentialed experts linking vaccines to serious side effects—including autism. Instead, Colbert blamed celebrities.

Offit has personally made millions of dollars from the development of a vaccine for rotavirus. Colbert made a joke of Offit being in "the pocket of Big Pharma" without telling us why.

Offit described outbreaks of communicable diseases that he claimed were ended by vaccines. Colbert brought up autism only to give Offit the opportunity to deny any link to vaccines. Neither Stephen Colbert nor Paul Offit showed any interest in what autism is doing to our children.

Offit cited twenty studies disproving a link to autism. Colbert never asked about the pharma ties that exist for every one of those studies.

Offit still can't figure out why 29 percent of Americans still believe in a link. (And he doesn't seem bothered by the fact that the higher the education level a parent has, the more likely they are to question vaccine-safety claims. It's college graduates aren't vaccinating their children.)

In the real world, parents are scared of a diagnosis that affects children everywhere that no doctor can prevent and that no health official cares about. Actually, Offit gave the audience the same arguments he's used for years. They've heard it all before, and it hasn't changed anything.

CHAPTER TEN

# THE REALLY BIG LIE ABOUT AUTISM

*"I won't be around forever. I want to know they're safe. I want to know there will be somebody to look after them, that they won't be forgotten and can lead productive lives."*

—Autism parent, *Kansas City Star,* Nov. 13, 2009

In August, 2006, I wrote a piece published on *Scoop.co.nz* called "The Really Big Lie About Autism."[1] The fact that there are so many false claims when it comes to autism might make it seem an impossible task to select the "really big lie," but I think I know what it is: Regardless of the stunning increases in the rate, no official is ever 100 percent certain that more children actually have autism.

Based on the theory that the public is more willing to accept totally illogical, absurd propaganda than a small lie, officials often tell us that all the autism everywhere is the simply the result of "better diagnosing" and "a broader definition." I wrote, "To be fair, while it's a lie for many, it's a fallacy, medical myth, or just wishful thinking for others."

The rate back in 2006 was one in every 166 children, and CDC officials couldn't explain it. Regardless, they weren't worried.

I wrote about how, when my son was first diagnosed back in 1993, I was told autism was "extremely rare" and that he was probably the only child in our little town of 14,000 who had the disorder.

Six months later, in February, 2007, I updated my "Really Big Lie" piece on *CounterPunch.org* because the CDC had just updated the official autism rate to one in every 150 US children.[2]

"The CDC announced this latest mind-boggling rate with an air of pride. CDC Director Dr. Julie Gerberding explained that the new numbers were because 'our estimates are becoming better and more consistent.'

"Now it seems that the CDC is on a par with the medical community with the news about this new autism rate. Not only are doctors better at diagnosing, but also CDC officials are better at counting.

"Incredibly, the CDC still cannot say with any certainty that autism is actually affecting more children despite all the autistic kids everywhere. The CDC has been studying autism numbers for more than ten years, yet they don't know if it's more prevalent.

"Dr. Gerberding explained it this way: 'We can't yet tell if there is a true increase in ASDs or if the changes are the result of our better studies.'

"The CDC still can't tell? This agency gets billions of tax dollars each year to run health care in the US. They can give us statistics on any other disorder or disease broken down by age, sex, and ethnicity, including changes in the incidence rate–except for autism. The study's lead author, Dr. Catherine Rice, made it clear that nothing in her research can tell us about trends. 'We hope these findings will build awareness,' Rice said."

Experts like Dr. Marshalyn Yeargin-Allsopp, chief of the CDC's developmental-disabilities program, and vaccine promoter Dr. Paul Offit were in the news telling us that autism really wasn't on the increase—it just looked that way. *ABC News* quoted Paul

Offit on February 22, 2007, saying, "People that we once called quirky or geeky or nerdy are now called autistic."[3]

The lie is regularly in the news. Reporters never challenge the doctors and health officials who tell it. It's been around for years and shows no signs of going away. It worked when the autism rate was one in 166, and it's been the claim with each subsequent increase in autism. What news sources reported in 2013, when the rate of one in fifty was announced, apply to any change in the rate.

*ABC News:* "Health officials say the new number doesn't mean autism is occurring more often. But it does suggest that doctors are diagnosing autism more frequently, especially in children with milder problems."[4]

*Fox News*: "'We've been underestimating' how common autism is, said Michael Rosanoff of Autism Speaks, an advocacy group. He believes the figure is at least 1 in 50."[5]

*WebMD:* "The main reason for the increase in the prevalence of autism appears to be better diagnoses, especially in older children."[6]

*USA Today*: "The higher numbers recorded in the new study suggest that officials are getting better at counting kids with autism—not that more have the condition, several experts said."[7]

*NBC News*: "The CDC says its new numbers don't necessarily mean autism is occurring more often, but it may indicate that it is being diagnosed more frequently than before."[8]

A mother interviewed by NBC: "I think it's scary. I think we obviously need to figure out what is going on."

Chief NBC science correspondent Robert Bazell: "But experts say the new numbers do not necessarily point to a genuine increase. . . ."

Dr. Zachary Warren, Vanderbilt University Medical Center: "Awareness is changing. . . . Clinicians are recognizing it much more frequently."

The Centers for Disease Control and Prevention has in recent years announced the update in the autism rate right before April—Autism Awareness Month. One might think that this would be cause for concern and that there would be a demand for answers.

Evidently not.

It's actually a very clever way to make the public aware of just how bad things are and, at the same time, downplay the results. Without exception, the major networks repeat the CDC's claim that it's not really an increase—just better, more accurate diagnostics. The point that was being missed here was that the CDC's claim of more accurate numbers when the rate was one in 50 was also used to describe the previous estimate of one every 88 children, one in every 54 boys, announced in 2012. And when the CDC backtracked to one in 68 in 2014, it was also better diagnosing.

The public has been conditioned to accept that, regardless of the jaw-dropping rate, there's never a real increase, and by now the numbers simply don't matter. The rate could be announced at one in 25, and news outlets would have still officials saying it was due to finally getting the numbers right.

The really big lie is the key to everything when it comes to autism. As long as the claim of no real increase works, autism will never be a crisis. If the autism rate is stagnant, then there is no link to the CDC's ever-expanding vaccination schedule. Dozens of top experts see nothing bad happening here. For the worried parent, it would seem that everything is under control.

The really big difference in media coverage of the autism numbers is between national stories like these and what's being said in local news reports. While federal health officials continue to scratch their collective heads, unable to determine if autism is a problem, it's a different story around the US.

Those who see the disaster coming and tell us about it can't give us a reasonable explanation. A news report from CBS on November 21, 2007, was typical.[9]

Anchor Harry Smith opened the segments by saying, "This morning, our special series on autism looks at a group of people you rarely hear about—adults. The adult population with autism is about to explode, as *Early Show* correspondent Maggie Rodriguez found out."

Rodriguez: "With so many children being diagnosed with autism today, it's only a matter of time before we're facing a crisis in adult services. At least that's what several experts are predicting. Right now, every child with autism in America is guaranteed services until the age of twenty-one. What happens next is called 'aging out,' when those services diminish, and all those now-adults with autism are left asking, 'What's next?'"

Rodriguez showed a young man folding laundry at a hotel in Chapel Hill, NC. She explained that he's autistic and isn't paid for his work but gains experience at a job. Unfortunately, she added, there may not be enough work for all the young adults with autism on the horizon.

Autism activist Alison Singer was covered, talking about "a tidal wave of people with autism" that we're unprepared for. She was adamant that America was not ready for "the one in 150 people who are going to need adult services."

Singer, who was described as the one of the people responsible for the establishment of Autism Speaks, the country's leading autism advocacy group, said that when autistic kids leave school, "they pretty much fall off the ledge."

Gary Mesibov, director of the TEACCH program at the University of North Carolina, was on camera next, telling the audience that despite all their efforts, they couldn't "meet this dramatic increase in need." He further said that programs for adults were the most difficult to fund and to maintain.

Rodriguez talked about the need for group homes to meet the need for the coming adults. She said that paying for them was "the biggest obstacle."

The segment ended with Rodriguez explaining the situation to Harry Smith. "The waiting lists are in the hundreds, they can't accommodate everyone, and there's not enough money to go around."

Smith quietly thanked Rodriguez for her report but had nothing to add. It's pretty obvious that the media simply isn't willing to honestly investigate why autism is a problem in the first place. Here lots of people agreed that there's a big problem coming that we're unable to handle. Not one person addressed the logical question: "Where are all these children coming from?" Why haven't we had to deal with this before? Members of the media cover this like disinterested observers who don't want to get involved.

Back on June 12, 2007, Harry Smith had an interesting column on the CBS News blog.[10] The title of his commentary was "Autism Can't Be Ignored." Smith talked about the 5,000 parents with claims of vaccine-induced autism in the federal vaccine court. He said that doctors had told him parents should keep vaccinating their children, but they continued to believe in the link. He called for more research, because, as Smith wrote, "The parents of autistic kids quite frankly don't trust what's been done so far.

And when people claim autism is just a new name for an old disorder, the press never corners those who try to convince us that there's no epidemic happening and that autism has always been around. Why can't they reassure us that there will be a place for these children? Why can't they show us the group homes filled with autistic adults right now?

Federal officials never waver from their positions of confusion and calm when it comes to autism. They can't tell us anything for sure about autism—except that vaccines don't cause it—but they're doing everything possible to address it, all the while it's nothing to worry about. They can afford to. Their job is to maintain the status quo. The real autism disaster will not affect them; it's going to hit the states. While the CDC is lost in the mystery of autism, the state governments will ultimately be responsible for caring for the victims. Do they even know the autism train wreck is coming? It seems unlikely. There's been too much complacency, and the clock is ticking.

On April 7, 2009, ABC News announced, "The Nation's First Adult Autism Clinic." It was all about a facility newly opened in California. The brief coverage disclosed a looming disaster that no one was alarmed about.[11]

The video segment presented the mother of a seventeen-year-old son with autism asking, "What do you know about a thirty-, forty-, fifty-year-old person who is diagnosed with autism? You never hear about it. The gap is obvious. There is no organized conversation about this topic."

ABC presented a pediatric neurologist who was starting a clinic for autistic young adults eighteen to twenty-one who were aging out of pediatric care. A voiceover said, "Most people with autism in California are three to eighteen years old, so the problem of addressing their needs as they become adults will only grow. Besides their medical needs, the cost of their social services is great, too. The California Department of Developmental Services says the state spent nearly $11,000 in 2007 on services for each child and young adult with autism.

"After age twenty-one, those costs more than triple when the state starts paying for food, shelter, and transportation expenses the parents used to pay for."

*TIME Magazine* had done something similar on Oct. 1, 2009, in a piece by Claudia Wallis called "For the First Time, a Census of Autistic Adults."[12] This was about the well-publicized research done in the UK that claimed to show that adults had an autism rate of 1 percent, similar to what we observe in children. Wallis announced the findings as conclusive. "On Sept. 22, England's National Health Service (NHS) released the first study of autism in the general adult population. The findings confirm the intuitive assumption: That ASD is just as common in adults as it is in children. Researchers at the University of Leicester, working with the NHS Information Center, found that roughly 1 in 100 adults are on the spectrum—the same rate found for children in England, Japan, Canada and, for that matter, New Jersey."

Wallis added that this study would seem to disprove "the commonplace idea that autism rates have exploded in the two decades." She said that researchers found the same one percent rate, regardless of the age of the adults. According to Dr. Terry Brugha, professor of psychiatry at the University of Leicester and lead author of the study, "I think what our survey suggests doesn't go with the idea that the prevalence is rising."

Anyone looking into the details of this research would hardly be convinced. Brugha found all the autistic adults by asking household members in Britain to agree or disagree with twenty survey items. These included things like: "I find it easy to make friends. I would rather go to a party than the library. I particularly enjoy reading fiction." After surveying 7,461 people from the 4,000 households selected at random, and narrowing the possible candidates down to 200, they found nineteen adults with ASD.

Wallis presented this study as proof that autism was nothing new and nothing to worry about. She also used it as further evidence that there is no link between vaccines and autism. "In England, where there is widespread suspicion that the childhood vaccine for measles, mumps and rubella has led to an explosion in autism cases, the study was hailed as part of a growing body of evidence that the vaccine, which was introduced in 1988, is not to blame."

To parents in the autism community, this was hardly evidence that society has always had autistic individuals around. It didn't make sense. Adults who were able to respond to survey questions had little resemblance to children who wander away, are nonverbal, rock endlessly and require care every waking hour. No one has ever been able to show us the adults on the severe end of the spectrum. No one is alarmed that they're not to be found.

KPBS in San Diego had a piece on November 12, 2009, called "Autistic Adults Present a Growing Care Dilemma."[13]

"The increasing number of Americans diagnosed with autism is partly due to an expanding definition of autism. But pediatrician Doris Trauner believes there has been a true increase in the numbers of people with this disability . . . the result of genetics, environment or a combination of both. We may not know what causes autism, but Trauner says the care dilemma that's caused by autism should be clear by now."

On November 13, 2009, the *Kansas City Star* published the piece "Adults with autism inspire worries and action," where they reported:

"Each year, tens of thousands of children diagnosed with autism, from mild to severe, enter adulthood and leave the safe confines of schools and their services behind."[14]

*The Star* said there was a "'silent tsunami' of autistic youth aging out into adulthood." Despite the fact that no one knows what causes autism, "the scope of its effects is vast."

In addition, one parent was quoted saying, "I won't be around forever. I want to know they're safe. I want to know there will be somebody to look after them, that they won't be forgotten and can lead productive lives."

In November 2009, "The Pennsylvania Autism Census Project Final Report" was made public.[15]

"According to the study, in 2005, there were close to 20,000 Pennsylvanians living with autism. Given trends, we expect that number to rise to at least 25,000 by 2010.

"The report also illustrates that the number of adults with autism will increase dramatically in the near future, growing by 179 percent to more than 3,800 in 2010 and to more than 10,000 by 2014."

"Things just aren't getting better, and individuals with autism are growing up. Now we need to include school-aged children, teenagers, and young adults in our mental snapshot. The number of autistic children expected to need extensive adult services by 2023—more than 380,000 people—is roughly equal to the population of Minneapolis. And, the bill for autistic children entering adulthood over the next fifteen years is an estimated $27 billion annually in current, non-inflation-adjusted dollars by the end of that period."

*Baltimore Sun* December 19, 2009, in the story "Autism found in nearly 1 percent of children," called autism a "public health crisis" and said that "750,000 children are now estimated to have an autism-spectrum disorder, and those children will be growing up to be adults and will need services throughout their life span."[16]

KING5 TV Seattle Dec. 29, aired World Within: Independence for adults with autism": "You know, we spend... the first twenty-one years of their lives getting our children ready to go out in the community; the reality is right now is our community is not ready for children like Alyssa. . . ."[17]

The *Washington Post* published the piece "Autism, not 'baby boomers,' biggest future health challenge" on May 18, 2010.[18] It was in a section on politics in Northern Virginia, and Richmond readers were given an ominous prediction: "The wave of aging 'baby boomers' needing public health services in Northern Virginia—once thought to be the greatest health care and fiscal threat facing local governments in the coming decades—will be far outnumbered by the skyrocketing percentage of young adults with autism diagnoses, Fairfax County Human Services officials said Tuesday."

*The Post* cited statistics from the Fairfax County Public Schools that showed their autism rate was one in every 83 students. This represented "an 846 percent growth since 1997."

Readers were told that Fairfax County was working with state and private agencies to come up with an adult day care program and that there was "a dire need" for all types of services.

There are no articles anywhere telling us about all the accommodations out there for autistic adults and all the services ready to meet their varied needs. How could the enlightened, humanitarian lawmakers of the last century have neglected this significant population? If autism has always been around like this, what did we do for the special needs of these adults?

In a story on June 20, 2010, in the Dayton, Ohio, *Daily News,* "Residency program offers activities, safe haven for adults with autism," the father of a twenty-six-year-old daughter with autism was quoted saying, "We're the parents that can't die."[19]

June 21, 2010, *ToledoNewsNow.com* published the piece "Parents worry about care for their adult children with autism."[20]

"One way to care for Ross as an adult is if he lived in a residential care facility or a group home, but spots at such places are scarce. In some cases, it is a ten-year wait to get in. This is because there are an estimated 27,000 adults with a developmental disability in the State of Ohio right now on a waitlist for funding to pay for their care.

"When Ross was diagnosed at the age of two, there were one in 10,000 cases of autism, but now it's one in every 110."

The Sunday newspaper supplement *Parade* examined what's ahead for young adults after high school on April 3, 2011, in the piece "Who Will Care for Dana?" *Parade's* Joanne Chen wrote about the future for hundreds of thousands of autistic children in America, and her story sounded nothing like what the British study purported to show.[21]

Chen described Dana Eisman, twenty, of Potomac, Maryland, as someone who "can't hold a conversation, make eye contact, verbalize her thoughts, cross the street alone, or control herself when she's upset."

Dana's parents said they were worried about what will happen when she leaves school at twenty-two.

"Support will dry up when the school year ends, leaving her parents to agonize about the quality of life their daughter is facing."

Dana was more fortunate than other children with autism because she does have an older sister, according to Chen. She's also been on the waiting list at a foundation that provides group homes for disabled adults since she was six. The downside was that the cost was "more than $70,000 a year, and those with the greatest need are served first."

Chen ended the story urging action to prepare for this population of disabled adults because "these issues are not going away." She said that more and more autistic adults will be coming, citing a rate of one in every 110 children, one in every 70 boys. Furthermore, the rate has been increasing 10 to 17 percent each year.

This was all very ominous sounding. Chen outlined the changes that would have to be made to accommodate this new population.

April 13, 2011, the *New York Times* talked about the coming adults with autism.[22] Reporter Amy Lennard Goehner called the task of meeting the needs of young adults "daunting," and she mentioned that Autism Speaks had come up with a "free Transition Toolkit" for parents of adolescents with autism. Parents need to plan now for their children's future. Geohner cited Autism Speaks' Peter Bell, who said that 500,000 young adults with autism would be aging out of school in the next decade. Nancy Thaler, executive director of the National Association of State Directors of Developmental Disabilities Services, was quoted saying, "The cohort of people who will need services—including aging baby boomers—is growing much faster than the cohort of working-age adults that provide care."

Goehner talked about group homes and "family-based care" as options for these young adults. With so many severely disabled individuals needing help, places in group homes will be limited. She predicted "long waiting lists" and presented the possibility that many autistic young adults could just stay in their family homes with relatives being paid to care for the autistic adult. A number of states are already doing this in some form.

There was nothing in the *Times* story to indicate that this was a coming crisis. After talking about hundreds of thousands of disabled young adults with no real place to go, the reporter advised that the simple solution would involve families providing for their needs. The obvious question of where are all the autistic adults are living at the moment never came up. One advocate said, "After Mom and Dad are no longer there, it is likely it will be the brothers and sisters who will ensure their sibling leads a dignified life, living and working in the community."

The idea that the US is going to somehow adjust to an increasing portion of the adult population in need of significant care seems like a lot of wishful thinking. For years, those directly connected to the problem in states all over the country have been saying just the opposite.

Fox 13, Salt Lake City, May 6, 2011: "A new study about autism in Utah presents startling numbers about how many children have been diagnosed with the disorder.[23]

"The University of Utah study looked at children previously diagnosed in Salt Lake, Davis, and Utah counties. It found that one in 77 eight-year-olds in Utah have some form of autism. That's double the number in 2002, when it was calculated at one in 154." A mother was quoted saying that no one knows what's causing autism.

The study's lead author, Dr. Judith Pinborough-Zimmerman, said she was aware there was an increase, but she was "surprised" to see that the numbers doubled in six years, and another mother asked what the rate would be in 2020 or 2030. She said we need "an air of tolerance and acceptance, and to realize that these kids are part of our community."

Oct 23, 2011, on CBS's *60 Minutes,* Lesley Stahl did several interviews about autism.[24] One was with neuroscientist Walt Schneider, and one was with Temple Grandin, an outstanding woman with high-functioning autism.

Dr. Schneider described a brain image of Grandin's brain as "interesting" and "a cool opportunity" to understand the brain better.

Lesley Stahl: "Do you see the day when you'll be able to say to a parent, 'Your child will never speak . . . so don't put all your energy into trying to teach them this. Put it into other ways for this child to communicate'?"

Schneider: "I see a day when we'll be able to say to a parent that there are multiple subtypes of autism. Your child looks like this subtype. And in other individuals of this subtype, they did or did not acquire language through various methods. . . ."

It was amazing to hear an expert so casually talking about children who don't speak. It was proof that autism has now changed our idea of childhood. Schneider talked about parents asking, "What really went wrong?" and going through "the grieving process."

Both Stahl and Schneider were at a loss to tell viewer anything of significance about autism, something affecting one percent of children and almost two percent of boys. Schneider admitted that parents are "desperately trying to find something that works," but he could only look for subtypes of a disorder that is now an epidemic far worse than polio ever was in the 1950s.

For those of us in the autism community who live with this disorder every day, the idea that there are subtypes is hardly anything new. Schneider can't tell parents why their child is autistic. He doesn't know what an expectant couple can do to prevent their upcoming baby from also ending up on the autism spectrum, and he can't explain why tens of thousands of parents report that their children were born healthy and were developing normally and that suddenly they stopped talking, lost learned skills, and ended up with a diagnosis of autism.

Schneider advised that parents have to go through "the grieving process" when a child is diagnosed with autism. Stahl acknowledges that some autistic children "will never speak." Neither of them expresses any real acknowledgement of what a nightmare autism has become for this country. One is left with the understanding that autism is now an acceptable part of childhood.

Stahl talked with Temple Grandin in an online segment called "Understanding Autism."

Lesley Stahl: "If there were ... a cure for autism tomorrow ... would you say, 'Wow! Give that to me!'?"

Temple Grandin: "No, I wouldn't, because I like the logical way that I think, and I wouldn't want to give that up."

Grandin and Stahl then speculated that it was an autistic person who made the first stone spear back in prehistoric times.

Temple Grandin is a well-known face of autism and because she's such an accomplished person, she offers parents hope. But she has little to do with what's happening to our children. Grandin herself admits that, in "a very mild amount," autism allows people to be successful. She's done well as an individual. Tens of thousands of parents, however, have children with autism who bear no resemblance to Temple Grandin. Many of these children don't talk. They're in severe pain from bowel disease. They live with seizures. Many are in diapers as teenagers and are in need of constant care because they're a danger to themselves and to others. And their parents are scared to death about how these children will live out their lives as adults in a world totally unprepared to care for the autism generation.

Grandin is from another era, when autism was rare. Autism is now an epidemic. If all autism were like Temple Grandin's, parents wouldn't be desperate to find answers.

While local press coverage tells us that fears about the autism numbers are real, the big news outlets continue to downplay what's happening. A month before the *60 Minutes* broadcast, on Nov. 30, 2011, *Forbes* carried the story "Living Life With Autism: Has Anything Really Changed?" by Alice G. Walton.[25] Walton wasn't worried about autism. She believes that autism has remained at a constant rate at the same time as she talked about the "fast-growing number of adults living with autism."

Walton wasn't alarmed about the 80–85 percent unemployment rate or "the estimated incremental cost per capita of autism is $3.2 million over a lifetime." Instead, her message was that we just need to create the right kinds of jobs for people with autism. She didn't dwell on the overwhelming needs of those with severe autism or express any concerns that the numbers might get even worse.

Walton acknowledged that "there aren't a lot of good statistics on how the work and living situations of [adults] on the autism spectrum have changed over the years." Why is that? Why don't we know what autistic adults are doing? She wasn't interested in looking for any of the 1.5 million autistic adults she claimed were out there somewhere.

Dec. 9, 2011, Walton followed up on her first *Forbes* story with "Living Life With Autism II: Perspectives."[26] In it, she focused on high-functioning adults who lately discovered they were autistic. She wrote about individuals like Ari Ne'eman, who serves on the Council on Disability and the Interagency Autism Coordinating Committee. She quoted Ne'eman saying, "Today people approach autism like some new thing that's totally unprecedented that we can get rid of. It's not new or novel, or a public health epidemic.

"We need to move from a vision of autism advocacy that wishes autistic people did not exist to one that includes us and where we enjoy the same rights and opportunities as anyone else."

Other adults were diagnosed in middle age, one at the same time her son was. She talked about Jonathan Elder Robison, autistic adult and author of *Look Me in the Eye* and *Be Different,* whom she described as someone who "has served on review boards for both NIH and CDC. He is a frequent speaker and commentator, and a long-time advocate."

According to Robison, autism is nothing new. "If we look back in time, autistic adults were doing all sorts of jobs, from composing music to engineering to working on the farm. Autistic people at all levels have been integrated. One might tend animals while another works with complex mathematics." He said that in the past, autistic adults "learned to fit in, and society learned to make a place for us."

Robison lamented the fact that in modern society, it was more difficult for someone with autism. "One hundred years ago, an autistic person might have learned the blacksmith trade, or learned to care for animals, and been very successful."

This attempt to explain away autism as a product of our modern society simply doesn't work. If autistic people were typically able to hold menial jobs or excel at technical ones, autism wouldn't be a crisis. Most autism parents can't envision their child simply blending into society at some level. They have children with serious needs, and they don't see these needs being met by the community.

In 2011, Alan Zarembo, at the *Los Angeles Times,* tried to convince readers that, despite the tsunami stories, there was nothing to worry about, in a four-part series called "Hidden in Plain Sight."[27]

Zarembo made the claim that experts just used to call autistic people something else, or they just missed them all together.

Dec. 11, 2011, "Autism rates have increased twentyfold in a generation, stirring parents' deepest fears and prompting a search for answers. But what if the upsurge is not what it appears to be?"

Dec. 16, 2011, "As more children are diagnosed with autism, researchers are trying to find unrecognized cases of the disorder in adults. The search for the missing millions is just beginning."

Zarembo explained that the epidemic increase in autism was due to a broadening of the definition. It was more of a "surge in diagnosis than in disease." He blamed genetics for all the autism. "The search for an environmental explanation for the rise has so far been fruitless."

Zarembo had experts to back him up. Roy Richard Grinker, an anthropologist at George Washington University, was quoted claiming there was only an "epidemic of discovery."

"Once we are primed to see something, we see it and wonder how we could have never seen it before."

Dr. Allen Frances, former chairman of psychiatry at the Duke University School of Medicine, said that it "makes no sense" to be worried about autism because "people don't change that fast. . . Labels do."

"Hidden in Plain Sight" was designed to put everyone's minds at ease. Readers learned, "Most experts see wider diagnosis—and increased spending—as progress. Children who in the past would have been overlooked, misunderstood or deemed hopeless cases are receiving help. But some of the same experts say that in the sweeping effort to find autism, some children are being mislabeled."

Lots of people were behind the explosion in autism, especially after the broadening of the definition in 1994. Zarembo believes that "a driving force" has been early identification of autism by parents, teachers, and doctors. Catherine Lord, director of the Institute for Brain Development at New York-Presbyterian Hospital and a leading authority on autism diagnosis, said, 'It used to be that autism was the diagnosis of last resort." Parents resisted the diagnosis. Now they prefer it. This is because having an autism diagnosis opens the door to "funded services."

Zarembo had even more good news. He cited a study from 2009 that found that 40 percent of children with autism lose their diagnosis. Even though autism is "officially a lifelong condition," research has shown that "it can be temporary."

Readers also learned that not only were better diagnosing and a broader definition behind the higher rate, part of it was because of over-diagnosing.

Zarembo cited Bryna Siegel, the head of the autism clinic at the Langley Porter Psychiatric Institute at UC San Francisco, who believes the radical shift in autism diagnosis has caused some children to be falsely diagnosed with the disorder.

"Mislabeling children can damage them psychologically and lead to wasteful spending," Bryna Siegel said.

To remove any doubt, Zarembo ended his series with an article where all the autistic adults are living. They've been right here all along. They would include those previously diagnosed with schizophrenia and mental retardation, along with those who lived in institutions. According to Zarembo, today adults with autism are living in "prisons, homeless shelters, and wherever else social misfits are clustered." But most of them are right here, in plain sight. "They live in households, sometimes alone, sometimes with the support of their parents, sometimes even with spouses. Many were bullied as children and still struggle to connect with others. Some managed to find jobs that fit their strengths and partners who understand them."

Zarembo claimed that based on "modern estimates," there were "about 2 million US adults" with some type of autism. He was confident that "society has long absorbed the emotional and financial toll, mostly without realizing it."

That last part about society being able to handle the cost and demands of autism must have been reassuring to many people trying to convince us that there is no epidemic and nothing to worry about. Still, no one had actually given us proof that the rate was the same for adults. Zarembo talked about adults with mild forms of autism who never received a diagnosis. The label of autism seemed to matter to him, but there is a bigger issue here. There are more and more kids out there severely affected by autism—Ones who can't communicate, can't behave, and can't learn. Regardless of what we would have called them, how is it that so many children were missed years ago? What did we do with them in a crowded classroom? Children having meltdowns, flapping their hands, rocking, spinning in circles—why weren't these symptoms discussed in the past?

And what about all the parents who report that their children were born healthy and were developing normally until around age two (coincidental to receiving vaccinations)? Suddenly they developed health problems like seizures and bowel disease. Many stopped talking and lost learned skills. Doctors are at a loss to explain this regression. Are we to just accept that bad things happen to kids?

The reporters who tell us that adults with autism are just as common as children with autism can't show us this adult population. I don't mean quirky-acting adults. I mean adults with the same signs of classic autism we see in so many of our children. Where are the head-banging, non-verbal sixty-year-olds in diapers? Where are the middle-aged autistic adults who have a history that includes a dramatic loss of skills as toddlers that were never recovered?

It seems the media will stop at nothing to convince us that what we see happening right before our eyes isn't what it seems. The real test of Zarembo's theory is the future cost to society as all these disabled children become adults. Will the taxpayers be able to handle all the better diagnosing?

Meanwhile the stories of jaw-dropping increases in the autism numbers keep appearing in news reports, along with stories about parents desperate over what will happen to their children as adults.

New Jersey has long held a leading position in the autism epidemic, and the press there talks about just how bad things really are.

Dec. 18, 2011, *NorthJersey.com* had the story "NJ autistic adults lack programs."[28]

"Many of those children, if not most, will need continued services as they grow into adulthood. And the programs for adults with autism are few and far between.

"'There's a tsunami of these kids coming, and there are not nearly enough programs,' said Carolyn Hayer, a Hackensack advocate for community programs whose son Chris is autistic. 'To invest all that special-education money in these kids and then leave them at home watching TV is criminal.'"

February 22, 2012, Fox 13, Salt Lake City: "Families of autistic children struggle to maintain heavy financial toll."[29]

"More and more children are being diagnosed with autism, and many families can't afford it. Experts say, with the numbers the way they are, more families will be seeking social services."

In April 2012, the president of Autism Speaks, Mark Roithmayr, had a *Huffington Post* piece entitled "Autism Is a National Epidemic That Needs a National Plan."[30] Roithmayr wanted action on several areas, including genetic and environmental causes, medicines, therapies, diagnosing, and training teachers, as well as addressing the needs of adults with autism. He called on Congress, the President, HHS Secretary Kathleen Sebelius, NIH director Francis Collins, and CDC director Thomas Frieden, to commit to such a plan. He ended the piece with a plea:

"This is a national emergency. We need a national plan."

While Autism Speaks may see the numbers and the inaction as a national emergency, the government does not. For years, every increase in the rate has been calmly announced by federal health officials who were still unsure that the new numbers really meant more kids have autism. No one at the CDC has ever expressed an interest in looking for an equivalent rate among adults. And no one in charge of health care is worried about where all the children with autism will end up someday.

Sept. 22, 2012, *Ventura County (CA) Star*: "California unprepared for wave of autistic children headed for adulthood."[31]

"In the mid-1990s, fewer than 5,000 people were receiving state-funded services in California for the developmental disability. Now that figure has reached about 60,000. The figure skyrocketed in Ventura County from a little more than 100 to 1,350.

"The average cost of serving an autistic person in the regional centers averaged almost $12,000 last year. The cost for adults has averaged in the $30,000 range, with half of the expenses for housing and day programs, according to the latest available figures from 2006."

A parent was quoted asking what lies ahead for the parent of a son with autism. Other parents had the same question. Yet another mother said she hoped that "perhaps her older son and relatives will help out after she dies."

Sept. 22, 2012, *NorthJersey.com*: "Of special interest is the growing number of children being diagnosed with autism—an estimated 1 in 49 in New Jersey—who are already a challenge to school officials. Jim Thebery, director of the county's division on disability services, points out that 80 percent of those with autism in New Jersey are under age twenty-one . . ."[32]

Oct. 2, 2012, *Cape Cod News* published the story "Parents plan campus for autistic adults."[33] The piece talked about "a 'tsunami' of people who have been diagnosed with autism in the last decade." Bob Jones, a parent, said, "We want a place for our son from now until he's a senior citizen." From his research on the Department of Education website, Jones had found that there are "282 kids with a diagnosis of autism who are now in the Cape and Islands schools." He was worried about what would happen to them as adults. Jones noted that when his son was diagnosed in 1988, the autism rate was "about one in 10,000." He said that by 2008, the rate was one in every 88, one in 54 among boys alone, according to

CDC officials. And he said the cost was concerning, estimated at "$90 billion annually, according to the Autism Society of America."

Oct. 4, 2012, the *San Francisco Chronicle* had an article that challenged everything Alan Zarembo said in the *LA Times*, "Experts brace for wave of autistic adults."[34]

". . . But he's also autistic, part of the generation of young adults who were born during the first big wave of autism cases in the United States two decades ago and are now struggling to strike out on their own.

"It was in the late 1980s and early 1990s that rates of autism started skyrocketing in the United States. A condition that once was considered rare, with fewer than 2 cases per 1,000 births in the United States, is now thought to afflict 1 in 88 children, according to the Centers for Disease Control and Prevention."

Supposedly it was unclear exactly what has caused the increase, but factors could include greater awareness and better diagnosing of the condition, as well as an actual rise in cases, perhaps related to environmental factors.

"It's not just a problem for the autistic children and adults, but for their families—especially for the parents, many of whom worry they won't be able to care for their adult children much longer."

Kurt Ohifs, executive director of Pacific Autism Center for Education in Santa Clara, talked about parents with young adult children with autism. He was quoted, "They come to me and say, 'I'm afraid to die, because who's going to care for my son or daughter?'"

So will we happily accept the autism epidemic among adults as these children age? Will taxpayers support the increases that will be necessary to support all the group homes and the services autistic adults will need?

If things continue like this, no questions asked, autism will become a fact of life for all age groups, and we won't remember a world where a significant part of the population wasn't autistic. The autism puzzle piece will become a common feature on stores, restaurants, and other places to show where people are trained to deal with those with ASD. We also have to remember, looking at the current rate, if one in every 88 Americans has autism, the other 87 are going to have to pay for that person. And if we accept that the costs can range from $3.2 million to $7 million per individual, the price tag will be huge.

Oct. 5, 2012 *Urbandale (Iowa) Patch*: "'Tsunami' of Autistic Adults Will Challenge Police; More Training."[35]

"'The tsunami of autistic adults is beginning to arrive. We'd better be ready, or we will continue to have tragic outcomes in these situations,' wrote Sherry Cook, a Lexington, Kentucky, parent of an autistic child . . ."

"'You can say it's more children being diagnosed. You can call it a tsunami or an epidemic, but nobody is really questioning that the CDC is wrong in their prevalence rate,' said Debbaudt, a Florida private investigator, whose son's diagnosis prompted him to form a company that specializes in training on autism."

Oct. 5, 2012, *Springfield (Missouri) News Star*: "New job program in Springfield prepares clients with autism"[36]

"Autism has become an increasingly used identification for determining eligibility for services under the Individuals with Disabilities Education Act. Meanwhile, the first wave of children diagnosed in large numbers with autism in the early 1990s is growing into adulthood."

Oct. 13, 2012, *The Orange County (California) Register*: "$255,000 raised at autism walk in Irvine."[37]

"With the passing of time, there are more autistic adults who need to find jobs, housing, and social opportunities like all adults," according to Phillip Hain, west region director of Autism Speaks. He has an adult son with the developmental disorder.

"'I am petrified for my son when he gets older,' says Sara Kelly, of Corona. 'He will be 200 pounds (when he's eighteen), and he's still having extreme outbursts. How am I going to handle that?'"

October 26, 2012, *Lexington (Massachusetts) Minuteman* had a piece in which a psychiatrist acknowledged the need for adult services while pretending that more adults actually have autism than children.[38]

"While the diagnostic criteria for autism-spectrum disorder continues to evolve, a generation of people diagnosed as children in the 1990s has grown into adulthood. With autism research primarily focused on children, adults on the autism spectrum are left with fewer options for health care services.

"'There are very few places in the country that take care of adults, even though there are more adults with autism than children with autism,' said Lurie Center Director Dr. Christopher McDougle."

McDougle was described as a clinical psychiatrist who has worked with autistic individuals for more than 25 years. Back when he started, the rate of autism was "only two to four people in every 10,000." And today, of course, it has risen to one in 88.

The only way this story makes any sense is if you totally accept that changes in the diagnosis account for the epidemic numbers of autism among children everywhere. Dr. McDougle said, "There are more adults with autism than children with autism." If that were really true, then there'd be no concern about all the coming adults with autism. They would go where autistic adults have always gone. The problem is no one has ever been able to show us the one in 88 adults with autism.

Feb 18, 2013, *Chicago Magazine* ran the story "When Autistic Children Are Children No More," where they called the coming adults with ASD "a looming tsunami."[39]

No one writing these stories ever wants to know why there aren't adequate services already in place for these young people aging out of school. And if there aren't middle-aged and elderly adults with autism living all around us, what does that say about autism? No one bothers to ask.

*Forbes* had more than one writer who has promoted the idea that there is no such thing as an epidemic of autism. September 25, 2013, Emily Willingham's story "Where Are All the Older Autistic People? Scotland, for Example" announced that there are lots of autistic adults out there.[40] There are people who would have had "diagnoses of 'mental retardation' in previous generations—labels that sometimes led to institutionalization—would be autism diagnoses today."

She claimed to have the science on her side to prove it and cited a survey done in Britain that supposedly found one percent of the adult population there with autism in 2009. To top that, she provided a link to a story in the *Scotsman* from September 23, 2013, entitled, "Older Scots with autism are 'invisible generation.'" The claim was backed by the National Autistic Society (NAS) Scotland urging the government to find these autistic adults who were "misdiagnosed by health workers." The *Scotsman* provided an example of how autism has been overlooked in the adult population. This was a sixty-seven-year-old man who had been misdiagnosed as "bipolar disorder and schizophrenia from his late twenties onwards." The individual described the social difficulties he had faced in his life.

Willingham had an earlier piece in *Discover Magazine* in July 2012 that also tried to make the case for no real increase in autism.[41] This one was called "Is Autism an 'Epidemic,' or Are We Just Noticing More People Who Have It?" and it coincided with the Centers for Disease Control and Prevention's announcement that the autism rate was now one in every 88 children in the US. She made it clear that if people start thinking there's really an epidemic going on, they look for what's behind it, or as Willingham put it, "The fear-mongering has led some enterprising folk to latch onto our nation's growing chemophobia and link the rise in autism to 'toxins' or other alleged insults. . ." Readers were told that the real reason for the update to one in 88 was the old, worn-out claim, used every time a new autism rate was announced: "Some researchers say that what we're really seeing is likely the upshot of more awareness about autism and ever-shifting diagnostic categories and criteria."

It may look like more kids have autism but, as Willingham wrote, "Autism is just a popular diagnosis *du jour* (along with ADHD) that parents and doctors use to explain plain-old bad behavior."

The medical community invented new labels like "Asperger's Syndrome" and "PDD-NOS," and suddenly there were a lot of people with the conditions, but they had always been here. Several times she emphasized that the supposed epidemic increase in autism was merely diagnostic substitution, greater awareness, and a broader definition of autism.

November 11, 2013, *the Times-Herald-Record* in Middletown, New York, published a story about federal legislation called the AGE-IN Act (The Assistance in Gaining Experience, Independence and Navigation Act), sponsored by Sen. Charles Schumer, D-N.Y., and Sen. Robert Menendez, D-N.J.[42] It would help those with autism transitioning from high school. The paper explained it, "To address the problem, Schumer introduced legislation that would provide funding to help organizations conduct research and aid young adults with their education, careers, and health care." Schumer was quoted saying, "Autism doesn't age out at twenty-two." Schumer explained that 50,000 young people with autism lose childhood services every year in America and that half of them don't get a job or go on to school. His bill called for research because, as the article said, "There's a lack of awareness of what services are available and most effective to help transitioning patients. More research is needed to develop techniques to address the problem."

Nov. 18, 2013, *Miami Herald:* "More than 80 percent of adults with autism between the ages of eighteen and thirty still live at home with their parents, and there is an 81 percent unemployment rate among adults with autism."[43]

There were other ominous signs starting to appear now. On February 11, 2014, the *Newtown (Connecticut) Bee* published a story that was a sign of the times.[44] The title, "For CT Adults With Developmental Disabilities, Housing Help Unlikely Until Parents Die," underscored the dire situation. There simply will not be funds for all these children as adults. The explanation had nothing to do with an epidemic of disabled children; in fact, there was no mention of the soaring population with autism as a specific problem. The lack of housing was due to of "the erosion of state funding for people with developmental disabilities" and "chronic underfunding." It seems that the state of Connecticut didn't realize that children with autism eventually become adults with autism.

Parents went to the state legislature to alert lawmakers to the critical need for help.

Among the examples of parents testifying was one mother who described her fifteen-year-old, severely disabled son as needing constant supervision.

Leslie M. Simoes, executive director of Arc Connecticut, was quoted saying that cutbacks to Developmental Services had resulted in "a time bomb waiting to go off."

While this story exposed the failure of officials to act, it had nothing about what was really happening or why it was happening.

More stories appear every day. On February 17, 2014, the *Worcester (Massachusetts) Telegram and Gazette* published something similar with "Autism After 22," in which readers were told that "the autism numbers are climbing" and that the state "is unprepared to assist the many autistic adults expected to need help with housing, self-care and other basics for decades."[45]

An expert was quoted saying, "The adult system, unequivocally, is not ready for the tide of autistic children aging into adulthood."

There are waiting lists, and it's estimated to take one or two decades before a place in a group home opens up in that state.

Incredibly, the piece never called this a crisis or recognized that autism is a whole new problem. The rate of autism was never mentioned. Toward the end was the simple line, "No one sees or reads about autism without puzzlement." The writer was happy to let officials get by with their failure to address this nightmare. And nothing was said about what's going to happen in Massachusetts when large numbers of parents die or are too elderly to care for these children. Will autistic adults simply end up on the street?

The really big mystery about autism is how we're going to pay for all the adults. It's obvious we have a problem. A lot of people talk about it but seem paralyzed when it comes to doing anything about it. Political commentators who complain about the "nanny state" and the "culture of entitlement" that has developed because of adults on federal disability rolls have no idea what's coming. Hundreds of thousands of young adults who never worked and paid into the system will be living off of it for a lifetime. We've had two decades in which we've done nothing about the soaring number of disabled children except to pretend it was normal and acceptable and leave it as a mystery we just can't figure out. Autism will now become an economic emergency. Maybe the cost of autism will finally force us to honestly and thoroughly address the cause of autism.

On February 22, 2014, the *Seattle Times* published a story with the headline "No funding available—A family's struggle."[46] The report described a broken system where 1,400 disabled children receive no help because there is no money available. Waiting lists were described as lasting from three to six years. The story focused on a boy named Rowan with severe autism but who received no services. The reporter never mentioned the exploding rate of autism and how this was a factor. Rowan was described as normal until he suddenly changed and developed autism. No further explanation was given.

What would be the reaction if this story were about blind children being denied services? Would officials be unconcerned if the headline read: "1,400 blind children receive no help in Washington"?

The people in charge seem untroubled when it's children with developmental disabilities. We're talking about children who often can't speak, who wander away and whose behavior makes them a danger to themselves and to others. The big worry here should be what's going to happen to all these children when they're adults and parents can no longer care for them.

I can't help but think of the play *Peter Pan* where Peter Pan lives with the Lost Boys on the island called Never Never Land, where they spend their never-ending childhood.

A lot of people pretend the children of the autism generation are like the characters in the play who stay young forever.

# Conclusion

This is a book I never thought I'd have to write. Ten years ago, when I began to send information to reporters covering autism, I had hope that things would change. I thought the ever-increasing number of affected children and the mounting evidence that autism is an environmentally triggered condition would force members of the press to report on it with a sense of urgency and thoroughness. That never happened. Incredibly, each increase in the rate was passed off as merely more "better recognition" of a disorder that's always been around. The media never questioned the validity of vaccine-safety claims from the agency that runs the vaccine program, nor did they look into the drug-industry ties of the experts who continually tell us vaccines are safe.

When I started doing this in 2004, the autism rate was one in every 166 children. As of 2013, it was one in every 50 children, including one in 31 among boys alone. Incredibly, officials have announced every stunning increase with the caveat that they're still not sure if more children actually have autism or if it continues to be "better diagnosing" by doctors and because, back in 1994, the definition of autism was expanded to included milder forms of the disorder.

When I first started doing this, I wrote right to reporters, hoping to get them to look into this topic. I sent links to studies, books and other information and urged them to talk to parents, organizations and experts to see for themselves what was happening. Rarely did I get a response. When I did, it was usually something like, "Thank you for your email. I'll keep it in my file in case I ever write on this topic again."

Members of the press don't see a real urgency in doing something about autism. Once a reporter wrote back to me and said that he'd like to do more on the topic, but his editor had "autism fatigue" because they'd already done four stories that month on autism. One reporter once told me that what I'd sent was very compelling but that I was talking about a conspiracy between government health officials, the vaccine makers, and the medical community, and there was too much oversight for that to happen.

Coverage about autism tends to show the public smiling kids interacting with teachers or playing on gym sets. In the three- or four-minute newscast segment we're told that autism is a disorder involving an inability at social interaction and a lack of communication skills. That doesn't come close to describing what thousands of affected children are like.

TV reporters and news anchors, along with big-name papers, never speculate on where all those undiagnosed, misdiagnosed autistic adults are. No one ever does the obvious investigative journalism that's called for here—namely, go to group homes and nursing homes where lots of disabled adults are and find the autistic ones. There have been false studies, most notably one in Britain, that supposedly have found the adults with autism. These were people who responded to survey questions about staying home alone or going out in social situations.

For two decades, news sources have told us that autism's cause is genetic. Endless studies looking for the elusive autism gene/genes are faithfully reported in the news. While there is speculation that there may be environmental factors, nothing is ever known for sure. There is lots of research on possible associations linking autism to older moms, older dads, even older grandparents, along with moms who smoke, drink, take anti-depressants, have bad antibodies, have babies too close together, and who live too close to freeways. These findings get a minimum of media attention, but, then, shortly, we're back to "autism's cause is a mystery."

Part of the conditioning of America to accept autism as just something that happens to some kids are the endless stories talking about fund-raisers for autism: walks for autism, bowling for autism, and lots more. The message "We need autism awareness and services." New parent groups, programs, and insurance coverage make it seem like everything's just fine. No one ever asks why there are so many stories about police, firefighters, EMTs, librarians, nurses, airline staff, and teachers being trained to deal with autism. It's common to find stories about "sensitive Santas" and autism-friendly movies and story times at the library in the news.

The reason I still continue to look at media coverage every day is because of the comment sections on these stories that appear on Google news on the internet. Reporters may not be interested in the information I post, but people read these comments. They can see that there are two sides to this debate.

If members of the press show no interest in the epidemic number of children afflicted with a disorder that no health official can reasonably explain, they're even less willing to cover the controversial link between vaccines and autism. It's much easier to quote a press release from the Centers for Disease Control and Prevention or a local doctor denying that vaccines cause autism.

It doesn't matter that many top experts do have serious concerns about vaccinations. All the studies by independent experts are quietly ignored. Hannah Poling and the 83 compensated cases of vaccine damage that included autism are never cited in stories about vaccines and autism.

This is the most heated controversy in pediatric medicine but it's universally presented as a debate between desperate, ignorant parents and mainstream medicine and public health officials. Dozens of peer-reviewed studies are never made public, but epidemiological studies showing no link do make the news. No one ever mentions that these population studies are the weakest kind of science because they're so easily flawed and the results manipulated.

The coverage on this topic is never fair, balanced, or thorough. The slant on most stories is to assure the public that nothing is wrong with having more and more children diagnosed with autism. The press has tried to convince us that officials have earnestly looked for a connection between vaccines and autism and that there just isn't one. If we can't trust the CDC and the AAP, who can we trust?

In 2009 and 2010, JB Handley, co-founder of Generation Rescue, wrote about something he called "The Hungry Lie." In the first piece, Handley quoted Dr. David Tayloe, then the president-elect of the American Academy of Pediatrics, repeating "the big, big, very hungry lie." In the words of Dr. Tayloe on *Larry King* Live, "Vaccines do not cause autism, and we're not afraid of the truth." Handley went on to cite other prominent people who've repeated "The Hungry Lie."

In his 2010 piece, Handley talked about another autism lie we're by now used to seeing in the news, namely that autism is a genetic disorder children are born with. Handley's hungry lies are closely tied to what I call the "Really Big Lie about Autism"—that there's been no real increase in the number of children with autism. If this lie works, then the link to vaccines is irrelevant because autism must have been around long before we were vaccinating children. And we don't have to worry about what's going to happen to all these kids when they age out of school, because we've always managed to provide for people like this—we just didn't call it "autism."

Handley was right: All the lies about autism are hungry lies. They have to be fed every day, which is why the media is constantly telling us about yet another study showing that vaccines don't cause our children to develop autism. It's also why experts cited in news reports never sound worried about autism or use the word "crisis" when talking about autism. That's why millions of dollars have gone into genetic research. They have to keep retelling the lies, or else people would wake up to the reality that there are a lot of sick children everywhere that no one can reasonably explain.

In the 1940s and 50s, images of doctors were used in ads promoting the benefits of smoking, despite a growing body of independent research showing the deadly effects of cigarettes. Today, the members of the medical community continue to appear in the news, assuring us that injecting known toxins into children and pregnant women couldn't possibly lead to the development of autism.

I am sure that all the lies about autism are on life support. There's a time limit to them. We're on the verge of an economic disaster as these children become dependent adults. It'll be the state budgets that will be affected most.

Good friends of mine in Minnesota have a sixteen-year-old son whose autism is severe. He's in a group home that costs the state $450 a day. That doesn't include his food, clothing or rent, social workers, or school. In addition, there are school costs that cover a one-on-one aide and total $30,000 a year. He lives in a group home with three other severely autistic boys—all the same age. The staff includes three adults during the day when the boys are home and one at night. His mother told me that the taxpayers will have paid out $1.6 million for his care by the time he's twenty-one.

This young man is the exception. Most autistic children, even the very affected ones, are living at home. The real autism crisis in this country will happen when these children become adults. Incredibly, we're doing nothing to prepare for this disaster, and it's a topic health officials are never asked about in interviews about autism.

The father of a severely affected nineteen-year-old girl I know told me that he asked the school staff what there would be for his daughter when she ages out of school in three years. And while they couldn't name any specific program, they were sure there'd be something for her when the time came.

What will there be for hundreds of thousands of these children after high school?

Why aren't preparations being made? The truth is no one sees any urgency when it comes to autism. If US health officials pass every stunning increase off as "better diagnosing" of a condition that's always been here, then no one has to do anything. It will be when the tsunami of disabled young adults descends on a welfare system totally unable to accommodate them that the truth will be undeniable. And all those who assured us for years that autism wasn't a really problem will have to tell us how we're going to provide for all the autistic adults who aren't here now.

# Afterword

*I would like to acknowledge that I could never have written this book without the years of experience I've had writing for the daily autism news blog,* Age of Autism. AoA *has given a voice to the autism community. Dan Olmsted is one of the many friends I now have because autism came into my life. I'm forever grateful that he asked me to write for* AoA *back in 2007. It's been an education. Here is Dan's story, in his own words.*

I first got involved with autism as a journalist in 2003, when I edited an article written by Mark Benjamin about conflicts of interest among CDC Vaccine Advisory Committee members. This, in turn, grew out of work Mark and I had done on an anti-malaria drug recommended by the CDC that had far more serious side effects than the CDC wanted to acknowledge. Because the drug worked, in the case of Lariat, the CDC seemed reluctant to look at problems it was causing, which included psychosis, suicide and violent behavior in US soldiers in Afghanistan and Iraq. That made us wonder if the CDC was also reluctant to look at problems, including autism, that the vaccine schedule may have been causing, according to thousands of parents and other eyewitnesses.

After Mark left UPI, I kept looking into autism and started writing a column, "The Age of Autism," in 2005. I was interested in the roots and rise of the disorder, and my research made pretty clear that autism was a new disorder, beginning with the first case series report in 1943. I followed these clues in more than 100 columns before leaving UPI in 2007.

With the encouragement and backing of the autism community, I started AOA later that year. Generation Rescue had just launched Rescue Post, run by Kim Stagliano, and, along with Mark Blaxill, we pooled our efforts to create *ageofautism.com*. Now, in 2014, we are still going strong, with wonderful contributing editors, readers, commenters, advertisers and sponsors. We call ourselves the daily web newspaper of the autism epidemic, and I also like to think of ourselves as the pirate radio station of the rebel alliance, giving voice and support to those who believe autism is an environmental illness, that kids can recover, and that the mainstream media and medical professions are wedded to outdated and self-interested explanations of autism as genetic—and never, ever linked to vaccines. Sadly, parents and a growing body of science say otherwise.

Dan Olmsted, Editor, *Age of Autism*

# Notes

## Unanswered Questions


1. Mary Holland, Louis Conte, Robert Krakow, and Lisa Colin, "Unanswered Questions from the Vaccine Injury Compensation Program: A Review of Compensated Cases of Vaccine-Induced Brain Injury," 28 *Pace Environmental Law Review* 480 (2011) Available at: http://digitalcommons.pace.edu/pelr/vol28/iss2/6.
2. Dr. Sarah Bridges, "EXCLUSIVE: Government Paid Millions to Vaccine-Injured Kids," Fox News, May 9, 2011, www.youtube.com/watch?v=tXp4hM3eQuI.
3. Mary Holland, Esq., "Law School Links Autism, Vaccines in Report," Fox News, May 10, 2011, http://video.foxnews.com/v/4687300/law-school-links-autism-vaccines-in-report/.
4. "Unanswered Questions" Press Conference, "Elizabeth Birt Center for Autism Law & Advocacy," Fox News, May 10, 2011, www.ebcala.org/areas-of-law/vaccine-law/unanswered-questions-press-conference-video.
5. Dr. Richard Deth, Heather McLennand, "Vaccine-autism link, New investigation," My Fox Boston, May 11, 2011, www.youtube.com/watch?v=Au4H24JwdUs.
6. "Possible Autism-Vaccine Link—Group says connection needs a closer look," CNN, May 11, 2011.
7. "Vaccines and Autism: Mixed Signals," Documentary, HDNet TV, August 19, 2011, http://blip.tv/hdnet-world-report/vaccines-and-autism-mixed-signals-5479546.

8. "New Study Reveals Autism Prevalence in South Korea Estimated to be 2.6 percent or 1 in 38 Children," AutismSpeaks.org, May 9, 2011, www.autismspeaks.org/about-us/press-releases/new-study-reveals-autism-prevalence-south-korea-estimated-be-26-or-1-38-chil.

## Andrew Wakefield

1. Karen D. Brown, "Parents Refusing Vaccines," *Boston Globe*, November 11, 2013, www.bostonglobe.com/lifestyle/health-wellness/2013/11/11/more-parents-are-refusing-immunizations-for-their-children-raising-fears-among-medical-community-disease-outbreaks/m3mGJgFhzrT7PUehai87tN/story.html.
2. Sharyl Attkisson, "Controversy Over Vaccine Research," CBS News, October 7, 2009. http://www.cbsnews.com/videos/controversy-over-vaccine-research/
3. Matt Lauer, "Dr. Paul Offit on *Dateline NBC* episode about Dr. Andrew Wakefield," *NBC Dateline*, Youtube.com, September 11, 2009, http://www.youtube.com/watch?v=hGrOS75I66g.
4. Matt Lauer, "Controversial autism doc: 'I'm not going away," NBC *Today Show*, May 24, 2010, http://www.today.com/id/37313063/ns/today-today_health/t/controversial-autism-doc-im-not-going-away/.
5. Manny Alvarez, MD, "Stop Lying About the Autism-Vaccine Link," Fox News, January 6, 2011, http://www.foxnews.com/health/2011/01/06/dr-manny-stop-lying-autism-vaccine-link/.
6. Sue Corrigan, "Former science chief: 'MMR fears coming true,'" UK *Daily Mail*, March 22, 2006, http://www.dailymail.co.uk/health/article-376203/Former-science-chief-MMR-fears-coming-true.html
7. Fiona Godlee, editor in chief, "Wakefield's article linking MMR vaccine and autism was fraudulent," *British Medical Journal*, January 6, 2011, http://www.bmj.com/content/342/bmj.c7452
8. Anderson Cooper, "Retracted autism study an 'elaborate fraud' British journal finds, CNN 360, January 5, 2011, http://ac360.blogs.cnn.com/2011/01/05/retracted-autism-study-an-elaborate-fraud-british-journal-finds/?hpt=ac_mid

9. Andrew Wakefield, MD, *Callous Disregard*, (New York: Skyhorse Publishing, 2010), http://www.skyhorsepublishing.com/book/?GCOI=60239100973200&
10. George Stephanopoulos, "Vaccine, Autism Link Called an 'Elaborate Fraud,' ABC News *Good Morning America*, January 17, 2011, http://abcnews.go.com/Video/playerIndex?id=12631458
11. Dan Childs, "Debate Rages Anew on Vaccine-Autism Link," ABC News, March 7, 2008, http://abcnews.go.com/Health/MindMoodNews/story?id=4402930&page=1.
12. Sharyl Attkisson, "The 'Open Question' On Vaccines and Autism," CBS News, May 12, 2008, http://www.cbsnews.com/news/the-open-question-on-vaccines-and-autism/
13. Wakefield, *op cit.*
14. Anne Dachel, "Dr. Halvorsen on Wakefield, Witch Hunts and Vaccine Safety," *Age of Autism*, February 8, 2011, http://www.ageofautism.com/2011/02/dr-halvorsen-on-wakefield-witch-hunts-and-vaccine-safety.html.
15. Wakefield, *op cit.*
16. Samar H. Ibrahim, *et al.*, "Incidence of Gastrointestinal Symptoms in Children With Autism: A Population-Based Study," Pediatrics, 2009, http://pediatrics.aappublications.org/content/124/2/680.full
17. Roni Caryn Rabin, "Regimens: Restrictive Diets May Not Be Appropriate for Children With Autism," *New York Times*, July 27, 2009, http://www.nytimes.com/2009/07/28/health/28autism.html?_r=0.
18. Kathleen Doheny, "GI Problems and Autism: No Link Found," *WebMD*, July 27, 2009, http://www.webmd.com/brain/autism/news/20090727/gi-problems-and-autism-no-link-found.
19. Nancy Snyderman, MD, "Autism Study: No Link to Gastrointestinal Disorders," NBC *Today Show*, http://www.today.com/id/26184891/vp/32168581#32168581
20. Robert Preidt, "Stomach Problems Common for Kids With Autism," *WebMD*, November 6, 2013, http://www.webmd.com/brain/autism/

news/20131106/stomach-troubles-common-for-kids-with-autism-study-confirms

21. "Children who have autism are far more likely to have tummy problems," UCHealth, November 6, 2013, http://health.universityofcalifornia.edu/2013/11/06/children-who-have-autism-far-more-likely-to-have-tummy-troubles/
22. Emily Willingham, "Blame Wakefield for Missed Autism-Gut Connection," *Forbes*, April 30, 2014, http://www.forbes.com/sites/emilywillingham/2014/04/30/blame-wakefield-for-missed-autism-gut-connection/.
23. Peter Lipson, MD, "Discredited Autism Researcher Chills Future Research," *Forbes*, May 2, 2014, http://www.forbes.com/sites/peterlipson/2014/05/02/1824/

## Hannah Poling

1. Sharyl Attkisson, "Vaccine Case: An Exception *or a* Precedent?" CBS News, March 6, 2008, http://www.cbsnews.com/news/vaccine-case-an-exception-or-a-precedent/
2. David Kirby, "Government Concedes Vaccine-Autism Case in Federal Court—Now What?, *Huffington Post*, February 25, 2008, http://www.huffingtonpost.com/david-kirby/government-concedes-vacci_b_88323.html
3. Jon S. Poling, MD, PhD, Richard E. Frye, MD PhD, John Shoffner, MD, Andrew W. Zimmerman, MD, "Developmental Regression and Mitochondrial Dysfunction in a Child With Autism," *Journal of Child Neurology*, doi: 10.1177/08830738060210021401 February 2006 vol. 21 no. 2 170-172, http://jcn.sagepub.com/content/21/2/170.abstract
4. Chris Cuomo, "Vaccines and Autism: Government Concedes Vaccine Case," ABC *Good Morning America*, March 7, 2008, http://www.youtube.com/watch?v=a5Ru-Tp27AM.
5. Claudia Wallis, "Case Study: Autism and Vaccines," *TIME Magazine*, March 10, 2008, http://content.time.com/time/health/article/0,8599,1721109,00.html

6. Sanjay Gupta, MD, "Vaccine case draws new attention to autism debate," CNN, March 7, 2008, http://www.cnn.com/2008/HEALTH/conditions/03/06/vaccines.autism/index.html#cnnSTCVideo
7. JoAnne Silberner, "Merck Hires Ex-CDC Chief Gerberding to Run Vaccines Unit," NPR, December 21, 2009, http://www.npr.org/blogs/health/2009/12/merck_hires_gerberding_to_run.html
8. Susan Todd, "New Jersey's Merck names new president of vaccine business," *NJ.com*, http://www.nj.com/business/index.ssf/2009/12/new_jerseys_merck_names_new_pr.html
9. "Former CDC head lands vaccine job at Merck," *Reuters*, December 21, 2009, http://www.reuters.com/article/2009/12/21/us-merck-gerberding-idUSTRE5BK2K520091221.
10. Sanjay Gupta, MD, "Unraveling the Mystery," CNN, April 4, 2008, http://www.cnnstudentnews.cnn.com/TRANSCRIPTS/0803/08/hcsg.01.html.
11. Paul Offit, MD, "Inoculated Against Facts," *New York Times*, March 31, 2008, http://www.nytimes.com/2008/03/31/opinion/31offit.html?_r=0.
12. Terry Poling, "Vaccines, Autism, and Our Daughter, Hannah," *New York Times*, April 5, 2008, http://query.nytimes.com/gst/fullpage.html?res=9400E6DC1F30F936A35757C0A96E9C8B63.
13. Sharyl Attkisson, "Vaccine Watch," CBS News blog, June 19, 2008, http://www.cbsnews.com/news/vaccine-watch-19-06-2008/.
14. Gardiner Harris, "Experts to Discuss One Puzzling Autism Case, as a Second Case Has Arisen," *New York Times*, June 28, 2008, http://www.nytimes.com/2008/06/28/health/28vaccine.html.
15. Dan Harris, "Gov't Examines Link Between Autism and Vaccines," ABC News, June 30, 2008, http://abcnews.go.com/GMA/story?id=5276589&page=1
16. Sharyl Attkisson, "Family to Receive $1.5 Million+ in First-Ever Vaccine-Autism Court Award," CBS News, September 10, 2008, http://www.cbsnews.com/news/family-to-receive-15m-plus-in-first-ever-vaccine-autism-court-award/

17. Alisyn Camerota, "Proof of Vaccine-Autism Link?" Fox News, September 12, 2010, http://video.foxnews.com/v/4336206/proof-of-vaccine-autism-link#sp=show-clips&v=4336206.
18. Margaret Dunkle, *Atlanta Journal Constitution*, August 12, 2008,
19. Margaret Dunkle, "We Don't Know Enough About Childhood Vaccines," *Baltimore Sun*, July 11, 2011.
20. Steven Salzberg, "The 'Baltimore Sun' Sinks Deep Into Anti-Vaccination Quicksand," *Forbes*, July 17, 2011, http://www.forbes.com/sites/stevensalzberg/2011/07/17/the-baltimore-sun-sinks-deep-into-anti-vaccination-quicksand/
21. Alisyn Camerota, "Damage from Child Vaccines: HHS Has Awarded Many Claims, Few for Autism," Fox News, September 19, 2010, http://www.youtube.com/watch?v=Sp5YWZVnpeI.
22. Lawrence Solomon, "Vaccines can't prevent measles outbreaks," *The National Post* (Canada), May 1, 2014, http://business.financialpost.com/2014/05/01/lawrence-solomon-vaccines-cant-prevent-measles-outbreaks/
23. Lawrence Solomon, "One-size-suits-all vaccines will soon be replaced by safer, more effective ones," The *National Post* (Canada), May 8, 2014, http://business.financialpost.com/2014/05/08/lawrence-solomon-vaccinomics-personal-vaccines/

## Sharyl Attkisson

1. "Sharyl Attkisson of CBS News has . . .," *CBS News,* June 22, 2008, http://www.ageofautism.com/2008/06/sharyl-attkisso.html
2. Sharyl Attkisson, "Vaccine Watch," *CBS News,* June 19, 2008, http://www.cbsnews.com/news/vaccine-watch-19-06-2008/
3. Sharyl Attkisson, "Learning from a Previous Vaccine-Autism Case?" *CBS News*, August 1, 2008, http://www.cbsnews.com/news/learning-from-a-previous-vaccine-autism-case/
4. Sharyl Attkisson, "Vaccines Linked to Autism?" *CBS News,* June 24, 2004, http://www.cbsnews.com/news/vaccine-links-to-autism/

5. Sharyl Attkisson, "Vaccines on Trial," *CBS News,* July 8, 2007, http://www.cbsnews.com/videos/vaccines-on-trial/
6. Sharyl Attkisson, "Healy on Vaccine-Autism Link," *CBS News,* July 28, 2008, http://www.cbsnews.com/videos/healy-on-vaccine-autism-link/
7. Sharyl Attkisson, "How Independent Are the Vaccine Defenders?" *CBS News,* July 25, 2008, http://www.cbsnews.com/news/how-independent-are-vaccine-defenders/
8. Kim Stagliano, "Vaccine Industry Group Calls on Couric and Attkisson for CBS Retraction," *Age of Autism,* July 31, 2008, http://www.ageofautism.com/2008/07/lisa-randall-of.html
9. Sharyl Attkisson, "The 'Independent' Voices of Vaccine Safety," *CBS News,* July 25, 2008, http://www.cbsnews.com/news/the-independent-voices-of-vaccine-safety/
10. "CBS News's Sharyl Attkisson Interviews Dr. Andrew Wakefield," *Age of Autism,* October 8, 2009, http://www.ageofautism.com/2009/10/cbs-newss-sharyl-attkisson-interviews-dr-andrew-wakefield.html
11. Sharyl Attkisson, "Vaccines, Autism and Brain Damage: What's in a name?" *CBS News,* September 14, 2010, http://www.cbsnews.com/news/vaccines-autism-and-brain-damage-whats-in-a-name/
12. Sharyl Attkisson, "Vaccines and autism: a new scientific review," *CBS News,* April 1, 2011, http://www.cbsnews.com/news/vaccines-and-autism-a-new-scientific-review/
13. "CBS Covers Court Award for DTaP (Whooping Cough Vaccine) Death," *Age of Autism,* January 20, 2011, http://www.ageofautism.com/2011/01/cbs-covers-court-award-for-dtap-whooping-cough-vaccine-death.html
14. Sharyl Attkisson, "Film provides glimpse into life of autistic teen killed by his mother," *CBS News,* August 30, 2013, http://www.cbsnews.com/news/film-provides-glimpse-into-life-of-autistic-teen-killed-by-his-mother/

15. Dylan Byers, "Sharyl Attkisson resigns from CBS News," *Politico.com*, March 10, 2014, http://www.politico.com/blogs/media/2014/03/sharyl-attkisson-to-leave-cbs-news-184836.html
16. Joe Coscarelli, "The Right's Favorite Mainstream Benghazi Reporter Resigns From CBS," *New York Magazine,* March 10, 2014, http://nymag.com/daily/intelligencer/2014/03/sharyl-attkisson-quits-cbs-because-benghazi.html
17. Howard Kurtz, "Sharyl Attkisson vs. CBS: Reporter first tried to quit a year ago," Fox News, March 13, 2014, http://www.foxnews.com/politics/2014/03/13/sharyl-attkisson-vs-cbs-reporter-first-tried-to-quit-year-ago/
18. Bill O'Reilly, "Sharyl Attkisson's career of investigative reporting," *Fox News*, April 10, 2014, http://www.foxnews.com/on-air/oreilly/2014/04/11/sharyl-attkissons-career-investigative-reporting
19. Brian Stelter, "Charges of bad journalism at CBS News," *CNN*, April 20, 2014, http://reliablesources.blogs.cnn.com/2014/04/20/charges-of-bad-journalism-at-cbs-news/

## Evidence of Harm/Deadly Immunity

1. David Kirby, *Evidence of Harm* (New York: St. Martin's Press, 2005) http://www.amazon.com/Evidence-Harm-Vaccines-Epidemic-Controversy/dp/0312326459.
2. Polly Morrice, "'Evidence of Harm': What Caused the Autism Epidemic?" *New York Times*, April 17, 2005, http://www.nytimes.com/2005/04/17/books/review/17MORRICE.html?pagewanted=print&position=&_r=0.
3. Gregory Mott, "Mercury Rising," *Evidence of Harm*, May 15, 2005, http://www.evidenceofharm.com/reviews.htm.
4. David Kirby, *Evidence of Harm,* http://www.evidenceofharm.com/reviews.htm.
5. "Evidence of Harm," *Publishers Weekly*, April 4, 2005, http://www.publishersweekly.com/978-0-312-32644-9.
6. David Kirby, *Evidence of Harm*, http://www.evidenceofharm.com/reviews.htm.

7. DavidKirbyCoaches.com, http://davidkirbycoaches.com/Book_Reviews.html
8. Don Imus, "Imus in the Morning," *MSNBC,* March 10, 2005.
9. Don Imus, "Imus in the Morning," *MSNBC,* April 4, 2005.
10. Don Imus, "Imus in the Morning," *MSNBC,* June 17, 2005.
11. "Vaccines & Autism" *Fox 5 News, New York,* February 14, 2005, http://www.authttp://www.autismmedia.org/media11.htmlismmedia.org/media11.html.
12. Jon Stewart, *The Daily Show*, Comedy Central, July 20, 2005, http://thedailyshow.cc.com/videos/uwf623/robert-f—kennedy—jr-.
13. Tim Russert, *Meet the Press*, NBC, August 7, 2005, http://www.nbcnews.com/id/8714275/ns/meet_the_press/t/transcript-august/.
14. Barry Nolan, "NiteBeat" *CN8* http://www.autismmedia.org/media11.html.
15. Joe Scarborough, "Scarborough Country," *NBC,* October 19, 2007, http://vaccineliberationarmy.com/2010/10/15/nbc-robert-f-kennedy-jr-vaccines-cause-autism-adhd-add/
16. David Kirby, "Vaccine-autism link?" *CNN*, March 6, 2008, http://www.autismmedia.org/media11.html
17. David Kirby, Jenny McCarthy, "Larry King Live," *CNN* (transcript), http://transcripts.cnn.com/TRANSCRIPTS/0804/02/lkl.01.html
18. Robert Kennedy, Jr., "RFK Jr's Autism Crusade Continues," *DemocraticUnderground.com*, http://www.democraticunderground.com/discuss/duboard.php?az=view_all&address=222x35721
19. Anne Dachel, "Autism coverage at the *NYT:* sins of omission," *Age of Autism,* April 18, 2008, http://www.ageofautism.com/2008/04/autism-coverage.html
20. Robert Kennedy, Jr, Boyd Haley, PhD, "RFK, Jr. and Dr. Boyd Haley Discuss Autism News," *Ring of Fire,* March 22, 2010, http://www.ringoffireradio.com/2010/03/rfk-jr-and-dr-boyd-haley-discuss-autism-news/
21. Kerry Lauerman, "Correcting our record," *Salon.com,* January 16, 2011, http://www.salon.com/2011/01/16/dangerous_immunity/

22. Seth Mnookin, "*Rolling Stone* re-posts RFK Jr. story lauding chemically castrating autism researchers," *Blogs.plos.org,* May 13, 2011, http://blogs.plos.org/thepanicvirus/2011/05/13/rolling-stone-re-posts-rfk-jr-story-lauding-chemically-castrating-autism-researchers/

## Generation Rescue

1. *JBHandley.com*
2. "Larry King Live," *JBHandley.com,* http://jbhandley.com/autism.html
3. ""The Doctors' on mandatory vaccines," The Doctors, *CBS*, December 3, 2008, http://www.bing.com/videos/search?q=barbara+loe+fisher+the+doctors+2008&FORM=VIRE1#view=detail&mid=61670F8FB46106A41FC361670F8FB46106A41FC3
4. "The Doctors," *JBHandley.com,* http://jbhandley.com/autism.html
5. *JB Handley.com*
6. *Ibid.*
7. *Ibid.*
8. *Ibid.*
9. *Ibid.*
10. Dr. Joseph Mercola, "The Smear Campaign They Used to Try to Shut Us Up," Mercola.com (video), http://articles.mercola.com/sites/articles/archive/2011/07/02/barbara-loe-fisher-on-jumbotron-ad-controversy-part-1.aspx
11. *Ibid.*
12. Matthew Herper, "Pediatrician Group Slams Delta Airlines for Running Video Made by Vaccine Skeptics," *Forbes*, November 7, 2011, http://www.forbes.com/sites/matthewherper/2011/11/07/pediatricians-group-slams-delta-airlines-for-running-video-made-by-vaccine-skeptics/
13. Barbara Loe Fisher, "NVIC Educates One Million Plus in Times Square on New Year's Eve, NVIC.org, http://www.nvic.org/NVIC-Vaccine-News/December-2011/NVIC-Educates-One-Million-Plus-in-Times-Square-on-.aspx

## "The Greater Good"

1. Leslie Manookian, Kendall Nelson, and Chris Pilaro, (2012), The Greater Good 2012, documentary], http://www.greatergoodmovie.org/
2. Anthony Kaufman, "Film Seeks to Spur 'Rational Discussion' on Vaccine Safety," *The Wall Street Journal,* April 3, 2011, http://blogs.wsj.com/speakeasy/2011/04/03/film-seeks-to-spur-rational-discussion-on-vaccine-safety/
3. Veronika Ferdman, "The Greater Good Review," *LA Weekly,* October 13, 2011, http://www.laweekly.com/2011-10-13/film-tv/the-greater-good-review/
4. Gary Goldstein, "Movie review: 'Greater Good,'" *Los Angeles Times*, October 14, 2011, http://articles.latimes.com/2011/oct/14/entertainment/la-et-capsules-greater-good20111014
5. John Anderson, "Review: 'The Greater Good,'" *Variety,* October 16, 2011, http://variety.com/2011/film/reviews/the-greater-good-1117946359/#
6. Jeannette Catsoulis, "The Fight Over Vaccines and Autism, Continued," *New York Times,* November 17, 2011, http://www.movies.nytimes.com/2011/11/18/movies/the-greater-good-review.html?_r=0
7. Jennifer Tuohy, "Pondering 'The Greater Good,'" *Idaho Mountain Express*, March 16, 2012, http://mtexpress.com/index2.php?ID=2005141182

## Celebrating Autism

1. S. Res. 78 (110th): A resolution designating April 2007 as "National Autism Awareness Month," March 23, 2007, https://www.govtrack.us/congress/bills/110/sres78
2. Secretary-General's Message for 2013, UN.org, http://www.un.org/en/events/autismday/2013/sgmessage.shtml
3. Emily Opilo, "Walk unites families touched by autism," *Morning Call*, Lehigh Valley, PA *http://articles.mcall.com/2013-04-20/news/mc-lehigh-valley-autism-walk-20130420_1_autism-speaks-autism-spectrum-sensory-processing-disorder*
4. Centers for Disease Control and Prevention Bottom of Form Autism Spectrum Disorder (ASD) "Autism Spectrum Disorder (ASD)"

Centers for Disease Control and Prevention, http://www.cdc.gov/ncbddd/autism/index.html

5. Harvey Kary, MD, "Cracking the Autism Riddle: Toxic Chemicals, A Serious Suspect in the Autism Outbreak," *Huffington Post,* http://www.huffingtonpost.com/harvey-karp/cracking-the-autism-riddl_b_221202.html
6. Anne Dachel, "The Really Big Lie About Autism," *Counterpunch,* February 27, 2007, http://www.counterpunch.org/2007/02/27/the-really-big-lie-about-autism/
7. *Ibid.*
8. Benedict Carey, "Study Puts Rate of Autism at 1 in 150 US Children," *New York Times*, Feb. 9, 2007, http://www.nytimes.com/2007/02/09/health/09autism.html
9. Dr. Catherine Rice, "1 in 110 children have autism, study finds," *NBC News*, December 12, 2009, http://www.nbcnews.com/id/34480829/ns/health-mental_health/t/children-have-autism-study-finds/
10. Miriam Falco, "CDC: US kids with autism up 78 percent in past decade," *CNN*, March 29, 2012, http://www.cnn.com/2012/03/29/health/autism/index.html
11. Michelle Miller, "More children being ID'd with autism: CDC," *CBS Evening News,* March 30, 2012, http://www.cbsnews.com/news/more-children-being-idd-with-autism-cdc/
12. Alan Zarembo, "Autism rates rising sharply, CDC reports," *Los Angeles Times,* March 30, 2012, http://articles.latimes.com/2012/mar/30/local/la-me-0330-autism-rates-20120330
13. Sharon Begley, "New high in US autism rates inspires renewed debate," *Reuters,* March 29, 2012, http://www.reuters.com/article/2012/03/29/us-autism-idUSBRE82S0P320120329
14. Lawrence Borges, MD, "CDC: 1 in 88 Kids Has Autism; Docs Debate Cause," ABC News, March 29, 2012, http://abcnews.go.com/Health/AutismNews/autism-rates-rise-88-cdc/story?id=16028834
15. David Brown, "Federal study estimates 1 in 88 children has symptoms of autism," *Washington Post,* March 29, 2012, http://

www.washingtonpost.com/national/health-science/federal-study-estimates-1-in-88-children-has-symptoms-of-autism/2012/03/29/gIQArD5XjS_story.html

16. Benedict Carey, "Diagnosis of Autism on the Rise, Report Says," *New York Times,* March 29, 2012, http://www.nytimes.com/2012/03/30/health/rate-of-autism-diagnoses-has-climbed-study-finds.html
17. Amy Harmon, "The Autism Wars," *New York Times*, April 7, 2012, http://www.nytimes.com/2012/04/08/sunday-review/the-autism-wars.html
18. Diane Sawyer, "Autism Increase Among Children," ABC News, March 29, 2012, http://abcnews.go.com/WNT/video/autism-increase-children-16034003
19. Mike Stobbe, "Better diagnosis, screening behind rise in autism," *Today.com*, March 29, 2012, http://www.today.com/id/46892046/ns/today-today_health/t/better-diagnosis-screening-behind-rise-autism/
20. Mike Stobbe, , "Health officials: 1 in 50 school kids have autism." Yahoo News, March 20, 2013, http://news.yahoo.com/health-officials-1-50-school-kids-autism-040223285.html
21. Steven Reinberg, "*US News* One in 50 School-Aged Children in US Has Autism: CDC," March 20, 2013, http://health.usnews.com/health-news/news/articles/2013/03/20/one-in-50-school-aged-children-in-us-has-autism-cdc
22. Rachel Pomerance, "One in 50 American kids has autism: What the latest figures tell us," *New York Daily News*, March 29, 2013, http://www.nydailynews.com/life-style/health/50-american-kids-autism-latest-figures-article-1.1302872
23. "Autism: One in 50 children in US have it, study says," CBS News, March 20, 2013, http://www.cbsnews.com/videos/autism-one-in-50-children-in-us-have-it-study-says/
24. Brian Williams, "Diagnosing Autism," *NBC Nightly News,* March 20, 2013, http://www.nbcnews.com/video/nightly-news/51264959/#51264959
25. "National Survey Pegs Autism Prevalence at 1 in 50 School-age Children," *Autism Speaks*, March 20, 2013, http://www.autismspeaks.

org/science/science-news/national-survey-pegs-autism-prevalence-1-50-school-age-children

26. Emily Willingham, "Autism Prevalence Is Now At 1 in 50 Children," *Forbes,* March 20, 2013, http://www.forbes.com/sites/emilywillingham/2013/03/20/autism-prevalence-is-now-at-1-in-50-children/
27. Jan Hoffman, "Parental Study Shows Rise in Autism Spectrum Cases," *New York Times*, March 20, 2013, http://www.nytimes.com/2013/03/21/health/parental-study-shows-rise-in-autism-spectrum-cases.html
28. Julie Steenhuysen, "US autism estimates climb to 1 in 50 school-age children," *Reuters,* March 20, 2013, http://www.reuters.com/article/2013/03/21/us-usa-autism-idUSBRE92K00C20130321
29. Karen Weintraub, "Autism rates soar, now affects 1 in 68 children," *USA Today,* March 27, 2014, http://www.usatoday.com/story/news/nation/2014/03/27/autism-rates-rise/6957815/
30. Miriam Falco, "Autism rates now 1 in 68 US children: CDC," March 28, 2014, http://www.cnn.com/2014/03/27/health/cdc-autism/index.html
31. Maggie Fox, "Autism Diagnoses Surge by 30 Percent in Kids, CDC Reports," NBC News, March 27, 2014, http://www.nbcnews.com/#/health/kids-health/autism-diagnoses-surge-30-percent-kids-cdc-reports-n63856
32. "CDC: 1 in 68 children diagnosed with autism," Fox News, March 27, 2014, http://www.foxnews.com/health/2014/03/27/cdc-1-in-68-children-diagnosed-with-autism/
33. Stacey Burling, "US autism rates up 30 percent in two years; N.J.'s is highest of states studied." *Philly.com,* March 29, 2014, http://articles.philly.com/2014-03-29/news/48666374_1_coleen-boyle-walter-zahorodny-jennifer-pinto-martin
34. "Dr. Walter Zahorodny Believes Vaccines Cause Autism," *Adventures in Autism,* April 3, 2012, http://adventuresinautism.blogspot.com/2012/04/dr-walter-zahorodny-believes-vaccines.html

35. "STUDY: Autism likely caused by abnormal brain growth during pregnancy, not vaccines," *ABC 7, Detroit,* March 27, 2014, http://www.wxyz.com/news/study-autism-likely-caused-by-abnormal-brain-growth-during-pregnancy-not-vaccines
36. Mark Roth, "Debate continues: Is autism really growing?" *Pittsburgh Post-Gazette*, October 6, 2013, http://www.post-gazette.com/news/science/2013/10/06/Debate-continues-Is-autism-really-growing/stories/201310060105
37. "Funding Autism Research," C-Span, August 5, 2009, http://www.c-span.org/video/?288235-1/funding-autism-research
38. Anne Dachel, "IACC Head Dr. Tom Insel Talks about Autism at MIT-Dec. 2009," *Age of Autism*, June 19, 2010, http://www.ageofautism.com/2010/06/iacc-head-dr-tom-insel-talks-about-autism-at-mitdec-2009.html
39. Anne Dachel, "Dr. Tom Insel on Autism: 'How We Prepare the Nation for a Million People Who May Need Significant Services,'" *Age of Autism*, May 19, 2010, http://www.ageofautism.com/2010/05/dr-tom-insel-on-autism-how-we-prepare-of-nation-for-a-million-people-who-may-need-significant-servic.html
40. "IACC Chairman Insel Testifies Before House Committee on the Combating Autism Act and the Accomplishments of the IACC," *IACC.HHS.Gov,* July 11, 2011, http://iacc.hhs.gov/news/news_updates/2011/news_2011_insel_congressional_testimony.shtml
41. "Autism Has High Costs to US Society," *Press Release, Harvard School of Public Health,* April 25, 2006, http://archive.sph.harvard.edu/press-releases/2006-releases/press04252006.html
42. "Senate Select committee on autism," April 28, 2009, https://www.youtube.com/watch?v=_dzj8a1jyMg&feature=player_embedded
43. "HHS Secretary Kathleen Sebelius Statement on National Autism Awareness Month," *HHS.Gov,* April 2, 2013, http://www.hhs.gov/news/press/2013pres/04/20130402a.html
44. Anne Dachel, "Kathleen Sebelius on Autism 'Awareness': Asleep at the Wheel?" *Age of Autism,* April 12, 2010.

45. Nick Meyer, "MIT Researcher's New Warning: At Today's Rate, Half of All US Children Will Be Autistic (by 2025)," *AltHealthWorks.com*, June 11, 2014. http://althealthworks.com/2494/mit-researchers-new-warning-at-todays-rate-1-in-2-children-will-be-autistic-by-2025/

## Admitting the Truth

1. John Larson, "The unorthodox practice of chelation," *NBC Dateline*, June 4, 2006, http://www.nbcnews.com/id/13102473/ns/dateline_nbc/t/unorthodox-practice-chelation/
2. Arthur Allen, "H1N1:The Report Card," *Reader's Digest*, March 2010, http://www.rd.com/health/wellness/h1n1-the-report-card/
3. "The Vaccine War," *PBS Frontline*, April 27, 2010, http://video.pbs.org/video/1479321646/
4. Neil Genzlinger, "Vaccinations: A Hot Debate Still Burning," *New York Times*, April 26, 2010, http://www.nytimes.com/2010/04/27/arts/television/27vaccine.html?_r=0
5. Jenny McCarthy, "*Frontline*'s 'The Vaccine War' Misses Half the Story," *Huffington Post*, April 28, 2010, http://www.huffingtonpost.com/jenny-mccarthy/ifrontlineis-the-vaccine_b_555785.html
6. Bill Moyers and Michael Winship, "When the Next Contagion Strikes—Vaccination Nation," *Counterpunch*, March 1, 2012, http://www.counterpunch.org/2012/03/01/vaccination-nation/
7. Robert MacNeil, Autism Now Series, *PBS*, April, 2011, http://www.pbs.org/newshour/spc/news/autism/
8. Anne Dachel, "The Truth About Liz Szabo and *USA Today* RE Autism," *Age of Autism*, July 3, 2012, http://www.ageofautism.com/2012/07/the-truth-about-liz-szabo-and-usa-today-re-autism-coverage.html
9. Liz Szabo, "With autism rising, researchers step up hunt for a cause," *USA Today*, April 2, 2012, http://usatoday30.usatoday.com/news/health/story/2012-04-20/autism-causes-researchers/53955958/1

10. Curtis Brainard, "Sticking with the truth," *Columbia Journalism Review,* May 1, 2013, http://www.cjr.org/feature/sticking_with_the_truth.php
11. Deborah Blum, "How the Media Fed the Anti-Vaccine Movement," *Knight Science Journalism at MIT,* May 9, 2013, http://ksj.mit.edu/tracker/2013/05/how-media-fed-anti-vaccine-movement
12. David Kroll, "Dr Paul Offit: 'Journalism Jail' for Faulty Medical Reporting," *Forbes,* March 29, 2014, http://www.forbes.com/sites/davidkroll/2014/03/29/dr-paul-offit-journalism-jail-for-false-equivalence-medical-reporting/
13. Association of Health Care Journalists, http://healthjournalism.org/
14. Emily Willingham, "Chili's Autism Awareness Problem," *Forbes,* April 5, 2014, http://www.forbes.com/sites/emilywillingham/2014/04/05/chilis-autism-awareness-problem/
15. Michael Hiltzik, "Chili's autism misstep and the downside of sloppy philanthropy," *Los Angeles Times,* April 7, 2014, http://www.latimes.com/business/hiltzik/la-fi-mh-chilis-autism-20140407-story.html
16. Katie Moisse, "Autism Community Clashes Over Cancelled Chili's Fundraiser," *ABC News,* April 7, 2014, http://abcnews.go.com/blogs/health/2014/04/07/autism-community-clashes-over-cancelled-chilis-fundraiser/
17. Jeffrey Kluger, "Chili's Burns Anti-Vaxxers: That's What Happens When You Kill and Maim Kids." *TIME*, April 7, 2014, http://time.com/#51612/vaccines-chilis-autism/
18. "Autism Speaks Announces Partnership with the National Autism Association to Provide Funding for "Big Red Safety Boxes" for Families of Individuals with Autism at Risk of Wandering," *Autism Speaks,* February 14, 2012, http://www.autismspeaks.org/about-us/press-releases/national-autism-association-big-red-safety-boxes-funding
19. Stephen Colbert, *The Colbert Report*, April 28, 2014, http://paul-offit.com/videos/

## The Really Big Lie about Autism


1. Anne Dachel, "The Really Big Lie About Autism," *Scoop.co.nz,* August 22, 2006, http://www.scoop.co.nz/stories/HL0608/S00224.htm
2. Anne Dachel, "The Really Big Lie About Autism," *Counterpunch,* February 27, 2007, http://www.counterpunch.org/2007/02/27/the-really-big-lie-about-autism/
3. John Stossel, Kristina Kendall, Patrick McMenamin, "Should Parents Worry About Vaccinating Their Children?" ABC News, February 22, 2007, http://abcnews.go.com/2020/Health/story?id=2892683
4. Mike Stobbe, "Autism More Common Than Thought," ABC News, March 20, 2013, http://abcnews.go.com/m/story?id=18768933
5. "Health officials: 1 in 50 school kids have autism," Fox News, March 20, 2013, http://www.foxnews.com/health/2013/03/20/health-officials-1-in-50-school-kids-have-autism/
6. Steven Reinberg, "1 in 50 School-Aged Children in US Has Autism," *WebMD,* March 20, 2013, http://www.webmd.com/brain/autism/news/20130320/one-in-50-school-aged-children-in-us-has-autism-cdc
7. Karen Weintraub, "Autism numbers rise in latest count," *USA Today*, March 20, 2013, http://www.usatoday.com/story/news/nation/2013/03/20/children-autism-frequency/2000131/
8. Robert Bazell, "One in 50 school children has autism," NBC News, March 20, 2013, http://www.nbcnews.com/video/nightly-news/51264959/ #51264959
9. Harry Smith, "Adults With Autism," CBS News, November 21, 2007, http://www.cbsnews.com/videos/adults-with-autism/
10. Harry Smith, "Autism Can't Be Ignored," CBS News, June 12, 2007, http://www.cbsnews.com/news/autism-cant-be-ignored/
11. "Nation's First Adult Autism Clinic," ABC News, April 7, 2009, http://abcnews.go.com/video/playerIndex?id=7279396
12. Claudia Wallis, "For the First Time, a Census of Autistic Adults," *TIME,* October 3, 2009, http://content.time.com/time/health/article/0,8599,1927415,00.html

13. Tom Fudge, "Autistic Adults Present A Growing Care Dilemma," *KPBS San Diego,* November 12, 2009, http://www.kpbs.org/news/2009/nov/12/autistic-adults-present-growing-care-dilemma/
14. Anne Dachel, "Autism and Adulthood, the Looming Future," *Age of Autism*, December 2, 2009, http://www.ageofautism.com/2009/12/autism-and-adulthood-the-looming-future.html
15. Anne Dachel, "Anne Dachel on the Rising Autism Numbers," *Age of Autism*, January 20, 2010, http://www.ageofautism.com/2010/01/anne-dachel-on-the-rising-autism-numbers.html
16. "Autism found in nearly 1 percent of children," *Baltimore Sun,* December 19, 2009, http://articles.baltimoresun.com/2009-12-19/health/bal-md.autism19dec19_1_autism-cdc-kennedy-krieger-institute
17. Jean Enersen, "The World Within: Unlocking the doors," *Seattle King 5,* December 29, 2009, http://www.king5.com/health/childrens-healthlink/A-World-Within-Unlocking-the-doors-79851912.html
18. Derek Kravitz , "Fairfax: Autism, not 'baby boomers,' biggest future health challenge," *Washington Post,* May 18, 2010, http://voices.washingtonpost.com/virginiapolitics/2010/05/fairfax_autism_not_baby_boomer.html
19. Josh Sweigart, "Residency program offers activities, safe haven for adults with autism," *Dayton Daily News,* June 20, 2010, http://www.daytondailynews.com/news/news/local/residency-program-offers-activities-safe-haven-f-1/nNDqL/
20. Melissa Voetsch, "Parents worry about care for their adult children with autism," *Toledo News Now*, June 21, 2010, http://www.toledonewsnow.com/story/12683793/parents-worry-about-care-for-their-adult-children-with-autism
21. JoAnne Chen, "Who Will Care For Dana?" *Parade Magazine,* April 3, 2011, http://parade.condenast.com/110577/joannechen/autisms-lost-generation/

22. Amy Lennard Goehner, "A Generation of Autism, Coming of Age," *New York Times,* April 13, 2011, http://www.nytimes.com/ref/health/healthguide/esn-autism-reporters.html
23. Anne Dachel, "Fox 13, Salt Lake City Reports on the Autism Nightmare to Come," *Age of Autism*, February 25, 2012, http://www.ageofautism.com/2012/02/fox13-news-salt-lake-city-reports-on-the-autism-nightmare-to-come.html
24. Lesley Stahl, "Apps for Autism," *CBS 60 Minutes,* October 23, 2011, http://www.cbsnews.com/videos/apps-for-autism/
25. Alice G. Walton, "Living Life With Autism: Has Anything Really Changed?" *Forbes*, November 11, 2011, http://www.forbes.com/sites/alicegwalton/2011/11/30/living-life-with-autism-asperger-has-anything-changed/
26. Alice G. Walton, "Living Life With Autism II: Perspectives," *Forbes*, December 9, 2011, http://www.forbes.com/sites/alicegwalton/2011/12/09/living-life-with-autism-ii-perspectives/
27. Alan Zarembo, "Hidden in Plain Sight Series," *Los Angeles Times*, December, 2011, http://www.latimes.com/local/autism/la-me-autism-day-four-html-htmlstory.html
28. Harvey Lipman, "NJ autistic adults lack programs," *NorthJersey.com,* December 18, 2011 http://www.northjersey.com/news/nj-autistic-adults-lack-programs-1.844445?page=all
29. Ashton Goodell, "Families of autistic children struggle to maintain heavy financial toll," *Fox 13 Salt Lake City,* February 22, 2012, http://fox13now.com/2012/02/22/families-of-autistic-children-struggle-to-maintain-heavy-financial-toll/
30. Mark Roithmayr, "Autism Is a National Epidemic That Needs a National Plan," *Huffington Post,* April 4, 2012, http://www.huffingtonpost.com/mark-roithmayr/autism-statistics_b_1403263.html
31. Kathleen Wilson, "California unprepared for wave of autistic children headed toward adulthood," *Ventura County Star,* September 22, 2012, http://www.vcstar.com/news/2012/sep/22/california-unprepared-for-wave-of-autistic/

32. Anne Dachel, "Hurricane Autism Has Made Landfall in America," *Age of Autism*, October 31, 2012, http://www.ageofautism.com/2012/10/hurricane-autism.html
33. K.C. Myers, "Parents plan campus for autistic adults," *Cape Cod (Massachusetts) Times*, October 2, 2012, http://www.capecodonline.com/apps/pbcs.dll/article?AID=/20121002/NEWS/210020339
34. Erin Allday, "Experts brace for wave of autistic adults," *San Francisco Chronicle*, October 4, 2012, http://www.sfgate.com/health/article/Experts-brace-for-wave-of-autistic-adults-3921071.php
35. Deb Belt, "'Tsunami' of Autistic Adults Will Challenge Police; More Training Needed Say Experts: Flashback," *UrbandalePatch.com*, October 5, 2012, http://urbandale.patch.com/groups/police-and-fire/p/tsunami-of-autistic-adults-will-challenge-police-more60147c740e
36. Ed Peaco, "New job program in Springfield prepares clients with autism," *Springfield (Missouri) News Star*, October 6, 2012, http://archive.news-leader.com/article/20121006/NEWS/310060006/Springfield%20autism%20job%20preparation
37. Ken Steinhardt, "$255,000 raised at autism walk in Irvine," *Orange County Register*, October 13, 2012, http://www.ocregister.com/articles/autism-374490-walk-speaks.html
38. Hannah McGoldrick, "Lexington's Lurie Center focuses on autism research and care," *Lexington (Massachusetts) Minuteman*, October 26, 2012, http://www.wickedlocal.com/x1660699788/Lexingtons-Lurie-Center-focuses-on-autism-research-and-care
39. Cassie Walker Burke, "When Autistic Children Are Children No More, *Chicago Magazine*, February 18, 2013, http://www.chicagomag.com/Chicago-Magazine/March-2013/When-Autistic-Children-Are-Children-No-More/
40. Emily Willingham, "Where Are All the Older Autistic People? Scotland, For Example," *Forbes*, September 25, 2013, http://www.forbes.com/sites/emilywillingham/2013/09/25/where-are-all-the-older-autistic-people-scotland-for-example/

41. Chris Valdez, "Schumer: Autism doesn't 'age out' at 22," *Middletown (New York) Times-Herald-Record,* November 11, 2013, http://www.recordonline.com/apps/pbcs.dll/article?AID=/20131127/NEWS/311270335
42. Christina Mayo, "Learn about autism at town hall meeting," *Miami Herald,* November 8, 2013, http://www.miamiherald.com/2013/11/08/3739775/learn-about-autism-at-town-hall.html
43. Arielle Levin Becker, "For CT Adults With Developmental Disabilities, Housing Help Unlikely Until Parents Die," *Newtown (Connecticut) Bee,* February 11, 2014, http://www.newtownbee.com/news/0001/11/30/ct-adults-developmental-disabilities-housing-help/190448
44. "Autism after Twenty-Two," *Worcester (Massachusetts) Telegram and Gazette,* February 17, 2014, http://www.telegram.com/article/20140217/NEWS/302179994/1020/mobile&TEMPLATE=MOBILE
45. Bettina Hansen, "'No funding available'—A family's struggle," *Seattle Times,* February 22, 2014, http://seattletimes.com/html/picturethis/2022957537_nofundingavailableafamilysstruggle.html

# Index